MATERIA MEDICA

OF

AMERICAN PROVINGS.

BY

C. HERING, M. D. W. WILLIAMSON, M. D.
J. JEANES, M. D. C. NEIDHARD, M. D.
C. B. MATTHEWS, M. D. S. DUBS, M. D.
C. BUTE, M. D.

CONTAINING THE PROVINGS OF

Aciaum benzoicum, Acidum fluoricum, Acidum oxalicum, Elaterium, Eupatorium perfoliatum, Kalmia latifolia, Lobelia inflata, Lobelia cardinalis, Podophyllum peltatum, Sanguinaria canadensis, and *Triosteum perfoliatum.*

COLLECTED AND ARRANGED

BY

The American Institute of Homœopathy.

WITH A REPERTORY,

BY

W. P. ESREY, M. D.

SECOND THOUSAND.

1853.

PHILADELPHIA:
PUBLISHED BY RADEMACHER & SHEEK,
No. 239 ARCH STREET.

MINUTES OF THE SESSIONS OF 1844 AND 1845.

"THE NEW YORK HOMŒOPATHIC PHYSICIANS' SOCIETY," in July, 1843, in view of the benefit to be derived from a mutual cultivation of the art by the various members of our school throughout the United States, appointed a committee to draft and send suitable invitations to them. They performed the duty assigned them, and on the 10th of April, 1844, a convention of the practitioners of Homœopathy of the United States, took place in the city of New York, at the Lyceum of Natural History, upon the anniversary of the birth of the illustrious Hahnemann.

Dr. CONSTANTINE HERING, of Philadelphia, was elected President; Dr. JOSIAH F. FLAGG, of Boston, Dr. WILLIAM CHANNING, of New York, Vice Presidents, and HENRY G. DUNNEL, Secretary.

A preamble and resolutions in these words were adopted, viz:

Whereas, a majority of the allœopathic physicians continue to deride and oppose the contributions to the materia medica that have been made by the Homœopathic School; and whereas, the state of the materia medica in both schools is such as imperatively to demand a more satisfactory arrangement and greater purity of observation, which can only be obtained by associate action on the part of those who seek diligently for truth alone; and, inasmuch as the state of the public information respecting the principles and practice of Homœopathy is so defective as to make it easy for mere pretenders to this very difficult branch of the healing art to acquire credit as proficients in the same;

Therefore, Resolved, That it is deemed expedient to establish a society entitled "The American Institute of Homœopathy:" and the following are declared to be the essential purposes of said Institute:

1st. The reformation and augmentation of the Materia Medica.

2d. The restraining of Physicians from pretending to be competent to practice Homœopathy who have not studied it in a careful and skilful manner.

Dr. John F. Gray was elected General Secretary of the Institute, and Dr. S. R. Kirby, Treasurer.

The Convention then adjourned.

First session of the "American Institute of Homœopathy" was organized immediately after the adjournment of the Convention on the evening of the 10th of April, 1844, at the call of the General Secretary elect.

Dr. Flagg, of Boston, was chosen, "viva voce," Chairman for the session.

On motion, the following named gentlemen were appointed the "Corresponding Committee" for the year 1844, and until the next annual meeting of the Institute: Drs. Clark, (of Maine,) Flagg, Okie, Taft, Cook, Fairchild, Gosewisch, Williamson, McManus, Pulte, Piper, Mose, Spalding, and Pilkin.

On motion, the following members were appointed the Publishing Committee, viz: Drs. Gray, Dunnel, and Kirby.

On motion, the following named gentlemen were constituted a Bureau for the augmentation and improvement of the Materia Medica: Doctors Hering, Lingen, Jeanes, Neidhard and Williamson.

The Institute then proceeded to elect, by open nomination, six boards of censors for the examination of future candidates for membership. The following named members were chosen, viz:

1st Board—Drs. Albus Rea, E. Clark, Jno. Merrill, all of Portland, Maine.

2d Board—Drs. J. F. Flagg, Charles Wild, L. Clark, F. Clark, and Wm. Wesselhoeft, all of Boston.

3d Board—Drs. Jno. F. Gray, William Channing, A. S. Ball, Abram D. Wilson, and H. G. Dunnel, all of New York city.

4th Board for western New York—Drs. Taylor of Rochester, Cator of Syracuse, Williams of Geneva, Robinson of Auburn, and Humphreys of Utica.

5th Board—Drs. Hering, Kitchen, Neidhard, Jeanes, and Green, of Philadelphia.

6th Board—Drs. Haynel and McManus, of Baltimore, and Piper of Washington.

Dr. A. G. Hull was elected Provisional Secretary.

Dr. Kirby moved that gentlemen of the profession whose names are not enrolled in the Institute, who wish to join it, can be enrolled by the Secretary, on their wish being made known, on or before the meeting of 1846.

On motion, adjourned to meet to-morrow at 11 o'clock, A. M.

April 11th—Met agreeably to adjournment at 11 o'clock, A. M., Dr Flagg in the Chair.

Dr. Hull presented a paper entitled "Homœopathy and Allœopathy contrasted, and a few of the causes which prevent the advance of true medical science, illustrated by cases in practice," by Geo. W. Cook, M. D., of Hudson, N. Y. (Referred to the Publishing Committee.)

Dr. Williamson, of Philadelphia, presented a paper on the "Podophyllum Peltatum," which being a new contribution to pure pathogenesis, was ordered to be read by the Secretary, and referred to the Central Bureau.

Dr. Paine, of Newburg, offered the following resolution: That in "the Homœopathic Examiner," this body recognises the firm and able advocate of Progress and Reform in medicine, and as therefore deserving the confidence and support of the fraternity of Homœopathists. (Unanimously adopted.)

Dr. Dufinel moved that the Publishing Committee be requested to address a circular letter to the friends of Homœopathy in the United States through the Committee of Correspondence, urging each one to become a subscriber to the Examiner.

Dr. Hering was elected a delegate to the general congress of Homœopathists to be held at Magdeburgh on the 10th of August next.

The Institute then adjourned to meet on the second Wednesday in May, 1845, in the city of New York.

John F. Gray, M. D.,
General Secretary.

Second Session of the " American Institute of Homœopathy," held in the city of New York, on Wednesday the 14th May, 1845.

The Secretary, Dr. Gray, called the Institute to order at 10 o'clock, A. M.

On motion, the body proceeded to elect by ballot a President for the session. The Secretary appointed Drs. Joslin and Okie tellers of the election, who reported Dr. Jeanes, of Philadelphia, duly elected.

On motion, it was Resolved, That the third session (1846) of the Institute be held in the city of New York.

On motion, the Institute proceeded to ballot for General Secretary for the ensuing year. The teller reported the election of Edward Bayard, M. D., of New York.

Dr. Snow, of New York, was then elected, "viva voce," Provisional Secretary.

The late General Secretary then read the minutes of the acts of the Convention last year, and also of the acts of the first session of the Institute, which were approved.

On motion, a committee of five, consisting of Drs. Gray and Joslin, of New York, Clark of Portland, Me., Williamson of Philadelphia, and Okie of Providence, were appointed a committee on "Constitution and By-Laws."

The report of the Committee on Finance was read and accepted, and on motion resolved, that the acts of the committee be confirmed.

The report of the Bureau for the augmentation and improvement of the Materia Medica, was then read, and, on motion of Dr. Gray, accepted, and the thanks of the Institute tendered to the committee for the zeal and ability which characterized the report.

On motion, Drs. Hering, Jeanes, Neidhard, Williamson, and Kitchen, were appointed the Central Bureau for the ensuing year.

On motion, it was Resolved, That a committee of three be appointed to ascertain the best mode of publishing the doings of the Institute, including the report of the Bureau, and Drs. Neidhard, Gray and Flagg were appointed.

Several communications were read by Dr. Gray, late Secretary, from Physicians, friends of the Institute, and of the science of Homœopathy, viz: Drs. J. C. Boardman of Trenton, N. J., J. Merrill of Portland, Me., J. H. Pulte of Cincinnati, George Lingen of Philadelphia, Adolphus Lippe of Carlisle, Pa., and Robert Wesselhoeft of Boston—ordered to be filed,

On motion of Dr. Dubs, a committee of three, consisting of Drs. Wells, McVickar, and Quin, was appointed on the subject of Posology.

Dr. S. R. Kirby was re-appointed Treasurer.

On motion, adjourned, to meet at 7 o'clock, P. M.

Wednesday Evening.

The meeting being called to order, it was

Resolved, That the vote making New York the next place of meeting of the Institute be reconsidered, and after considerable discussion it was

Resolved, That the next meeting of the Institute be held in Philadelphia on the second Wednesday of May, 1846.

Resolved, That Docts. Bayard, Gray, and Cook, be a committee for the purpose of engrossing the 1st vol. of the Transactions of the Institute, and superintending the publication of the same, and that the Central Bureau be requested to co-operate with the committee in the publication.

The committee appointed to nominate a board of censors, reported in favor of re-appointing the members of the several boards of the last session to constitute one board, and that any three censors may constitute a board for the examination of candidates and a recommendation of a majority of said board shall render a candidate eligible to membership in this Institute, which was adopted.

Adjourned to meet to-morrow morning at 10 o'clock.

Thursday Morning, May 15th, 1845.

The meeting was called to order by the President, and the minutes of last meeting read and approved.

On motion, *Resolved*, That the Secretary be instructed to procure a suitable seal for the Institute.

On motion, *Resolved*, That the Publishing Committee prepare a report of the proceedings of the Institute, to be published in several newspapers, and that each member be served with a copy of the same.

On motion, *Resolved*, Not to admit as a member of this Institute, any person who has not pursued a regular course of medical studies according to the requirements of the existing medical institutions of our country, and, in addition thereto, sustained an examination before the censors of this Institute on the theory and practice of Homœopathy.

Adjourned to meet at 8 o'clock this evening.

Thursday Evening.

The President called the meeting to order; minutes of last meeting read and approved.

On motion of Dr. Gray, *Resolved*, That the Bureau for the augmentation and improvement of the Materia Medica, be earnestly solicited to deliberate and report upon a scientific arrangement of the Materia Medica at the next session of the Institute.

On motion, *Resolved*, That a committee of five be appointed to frame and procure certificates of ordinary and honorary membership to be furnished to members at such a price as the committee shall determine. Docts. Bayard, Quin, Gray, Hempel and Joslin were appointed.

Resolved, That the statute appointing a committee of correspondence be annulled.

Resolved, That Constantine Hering, M. D., of Philadelphia, be appointed a delegate to represent the American Institute of Homœopathy in the Congress of Homœopathists to be held in Germany on the 10th day of August next.

Resolved, That the thanks of the Institute be tendered to Dr. Jeanes, for the able manner in which he has discharged the duties of chairman of the Institute.

On motion the Convention adjourned to meet again at Philadelphia on the second Wednesday of May, 1846, at 10 o'clock, A. M.

EDWARD BAYARD, M. D.,
Gen. Secretary.

INTRODUCTORY REPORT

OF

THE CENTRAL BUREAU.

At the first meeting of the American Institute of Homœopathy, held in the city of New York, in April, 1844, a Committee was appointed entitled the "Central Bureau," for the augmentation and improvement of the Materia Medica.

Sensible of the importance of the trust committed, it immediately made arrangements to secure the co-operation of Homœopathists generally.

A circular was addressed to all the Homœopathic Physicians of this country, at that time known to it, soliciting information on three topics, viz.:

"1st. The effects which you have observed from remedies not mentioned in Jahr's Manual, whether in health or disease; stating the precise localities of the symptoms, the times of the day at which they occurred, with all the attending circumstances.

"2d. New symptoms, either pathogenetic or curative which you may have observed from the remedies in Jahr's Manual, which are clearly ascribable to those remedies, with the particulars of each case.

"3d. The symptoms which you have seen confirmed most frequently in your practice; also, any remarkable coincidences in allœopathic or popular practice, and especially cases of poisoning, which may have come under your observation."

In the circular, three new remedies were also proposed for trial, viz.: Oxalic acid, Podophyllum peltatum and Kalmia latifolia, and an offer made to furnish all of them to all who should apply. A number of applications were received, and the medicines sent accordingly.

The Bureau has also received communications from the following gentlemen, relating cases of cure or requesting medicines for experimentation: Dr. G. W. Swazey, of Springfield, Massachusetts; J. Merrill, Portland, Maine; D. S. Kimball, Sacket's Harbor, New York; Joel Divine, Poughkeepsie, New York; T. Percival Royston, Lockport, New York; J. C. Boardman, Trenton, New Jersey; Josiah F. Flagg, Boston.

The work of elaborating the Report was performed as follows:

Benzoic acid, tried and arranged by Dr. Jacob Jeanes, with contributions of symptoms from Dr. Lingen.

Eupatorium perfoliatum, tried and arranged by Dr. Williamson, with contributions of symptoms from Dr. Neidhard.

Fluoric acid, tried and arranged by Dr. Hering, with contributions of symptoms from Drs. Campos, Lippe, Jeanes, Neidhard, Williamson, Husmann, Pehrson, Freytag, Gosewisch, Geist, and Messrs. Smith and Behlert.

Kalmia latifolia, tried and arranged by Dr. Hering, with contributions of symptoms from Drs. Freytag, Bauer, Schmidt, Williamson, Fairchild, E. Clark, and Mr. Behlert.

Lobelia cardinalis, tried by Dr. Dubs.

Lobelia inflata, tried and arranged by Dr. Jeanes, with contributions of symptoms from Drs. Williamson, Geist, Gosewisch, and also with the aid of the treatise by Dr. Noack, of Leipsic.

Oxalic acid, tried and arranged by Dr. Neidhard, with contributions of symptoms from Drs. Hering, Floto, Smith, Dubs, Kitchen and Williamson.

Podophyllum peltatum, tried and arranged by Dr. Williamson, with contributions of symptoms from Drs. Jeanes, Ward, Husmann, Hering and Fairchild.

Sanguinaria canadensis, tried by Dr. Bute, with contributions of symptoms from Drs. Hering, Husmann, Jeanes, Neidhard and Mr. Behlert.

Triosteum perfoliatum, tried by Dr. Williamson, with contributions of symptoms from Dr. Neidhard.

The Bureau is indebted to Dr. William P. Esrey, for the valuable addition of the Repertorium.

There are several matters which may be thought to require either apology or defence. A brief notice of a few of them is esteemed necessary.

The first in importance, especially as it was embraced in the duties of the Central Bureau, is that no new or improved arrangement of the materia medica has been performed or even attempted; and the only apology which can be offered for this neglect is, that the means for accomplishing this task are as yet insufficient. To increase those means, has been an ardent desire of the Bureau, and it has not failed to labor for the furtherance of this object. At an early date from its creation, it addressed a circular to all the Homœopathic Physicians on this continent, who were at that time known to it, requesting of them statements of confirmed symptoms, &c., a species of knowledge which is absolutely indispensable in a proper re-arrangement of the materia medica.

This request has met with so faint a response from the profession in general, that as yet the means under the control of the Bureau are not much increased. But it is hoped that the necessity of this knowledge will soon be seen and felt not only in this country but throughout the world, and that every physician will hasten to cast his tribute, though only a mite, into the treasury of knowledge; and we anticipate with pleasure that the physicians of this country will yet be in advance in the good work. The following defence of other points will aid in bringing into view the positive need which exists for this united labour of physicians for the advancement of the healing art.

It may be objected to the report, that the Bureau has thrown into the materia medica fragmentary observations upon half a dozen or more remedies which are new to it; adding to the already cumbersome mass of imperfectly understood medicines without materially advancing the science.

To answer this objection to the satisfaction of those who think a remedy to be known in proportion to the number of symptoms which have been attributed to it, would be extremely difficult, if not impossible. But others can understand, that a remedy of which we know one positive group of symptoms corresponding to similar groups, in diseases of frequent occurrence, may be a more valuable remedy, and better known with twenty symptoms, than another medicine with hundreds of symptoms, but of which we know with certainty of no groups in which they are particularly applicable. To fully appreciate the correctness of these remarks, a cursory glance of our materia medica is only required, with the additional observation of the fact that we have but few publications of cases cured by some remedies, which, from their extensive list of symptoms, would appear to have been largely experimented upon. It is true, that they may have been more extensively and advantageously employed than would be supposed. But if this be the fact it is high time that it were known.

The Bureau might adduce the authority of Hahnemann for the propriety and necessity of investigating the properties of new remedies. Both observation and experience combine to show that no one remedy will suffice to cure a thousandth part of the diseases to which man is subject. That when a succession of remedies has been required to cure a complaint in one instance, the discovery of a remedy more adapted has led to the immediate cure of very similar disorders. And from this it may be inferred that, with all possible accurate knowledge of the properties of remedies, an extensive materia medica will be requisite to meet and conquer the multitudinous diseases with which mankind is afflicted. But to render such a materia medica fully available, there must be condensation. The strong symptoms, not merely the most violent, but those of most frequent occurrence, must be known. The true must be separated from the doubtful and the false. Cut out these from our list of symptoms, and these lists will be abridged. Put together in one place a symptom which is variously expressed and now appears as a variety of symptoms, and we have valuable condensation. But these are not light and easy works, readily to be accomplished. The path we have travelled was the necessary one. It is a necessary one in regard to every new remedy; we must accept the symptoms which follow its trial as its effects, and so set them down. If this were not done there could be no beginning, and without a beginning there could have been no progress. But that we should always continue to acknowledge as positive effects of a remedy those symptoms which occurred to an experimenter after a trial of medicine, though these have been confirmed by no other experimenter, is the height of absurdity. Therefore the Bureau again urges the profession to come forward to the work of ascertaining the most positive of the symptoms of remedies.

CONSTANTINE HERING, M. D.
JACOB JEANES, M. D.
CHARLES NEIDHARD, M. D.
WALTER WILLIAMSON, M. D.
JAMES KITCHEN, M. D.

REPORT OF THE CENTRAL BUREAU.

ACIDUM BENZOICUM.

BY JACOB JEANES, M. D.

Benzoic Acid. Flowers of Benzoin. Germ. Benzoeblumen. Benzoesalz.

THE benzoic acid derives its name from the gum benzoin or benjamin, which is the concrete juice of a tree, the Styrax benzoin, a native of Sumatra, Java, Laos and Siam.

Though this acid is found most abundantly in the benzoin, yet it also exists in the dragon's blood, in the anthoxanthum odoratum and holcus odoratus. Its presence in other plants is doubtful; in storax, peruvian balsam, cinnamon and cinnamon oil, it is the cinnamomic acid which has been mistaken for it. It has also been stated to exist in the urine of herbivorous quadrupeds, forming on the average, as stated by Vauquelin, about one three-hundredths of the urine of this class of animals. But according to Liebig, this is hippuric and not benzoic acid. The oil of bitter almonds is converted into benzoic acid, simply by the addition of oxygen.

For pharmaceutical use, it is directed by the United States, London, Edinburgh and Dublin Pharmocopœias, that the benzoic acid should be procured from the gum benzoin. It is obtained either by sublimation or by dissolving the gum in alkaline waters, then decomposing the benzoates thus formed, by the addition of an acid, and afterwards purifying the benzoic acid thus precipitated, by washing it with cold water, which dissolves but one four-hundreth of its weight of the acid, whilst boiling water dissolves one-twentieth. The process of obtaining the benzoic acid by sublimation is directed by the United States and London Pharmacopœias, and the acid thus procured is, for various reasons, that which is to be preferred for medicinal use.

Benzoic acid contains 69.25 per cent. of carbon, 4.86 of hydrogen, and 25.89 of oxygen; or, as stated by Liebig, it is composed of 14 equivalents of carbon, 10 of hydrogen and 3 of oxygen.

This acid was described as long since as 1608, by Blaise de Bigenere, under the name of Flowers of Benzoin.

In medicine it has been employed in two preparations known by the name of paregoric elixir, viz: the Tinctura Opii Camphorata and the Tinctura Opii Ammoniata of the dispensatories. In the latter preparation it must form benzoate of ammonia instead of existing in the form of a free acid.

Although these tinctures have been extensively and for a long time employed by physicians, yet none of the writers on the materia medica appear disposed to attribute any medicinal power to the benzoic acid; and most who speak on the subject appear to concur with Murray, who remarks that "it has been regarded as a stimulating expectorant, but is totally destitute of medicinal efficacy, and the sole consumption of it is in the composition of the paregoric elixirs of the pharmacopœias, in which, as it has long been an ingredient, it is still retained."

Eight years ago I instituted experiments with the view to ascertain the effects of this acid on the human body in a state of health; and several symptoms then observed have since been repeatedly confirmed in persons who had taken the tinctura opii camphorata.

Guided by the information thus acquired, to its employment as an agent for the removal of disease, I was forcibly struck by the power which it exerted in altering the secretory action of the kidneys, in many cases where the urine was of a deep red color, and yielded an uncommonly strong urinous odor.

About four years since, Dr. Alexander Ure recommended the benzoic acid as a remedy which he believed to be likely to prevent the formation of tophous secretions in gouty subjects. He administered it in doses of a scruple, an hour after a meal. In the course of a couple of hours the urine voided, amounting to five or six ounces, yielded, on the addition of a twelfth part of muriatic acid, a copious precipitate of beautiful rose-pink acicular crystals, precisely the crystalline character of an acid peculiar to graminivrous animals, and to which Liebig has assigned the name of hippuric acid. In the urine, after the benzoic acid, the hippuric acid was found to have taken the place of the uric acid, none of the latter being discoverable.

As the salts formed by the combination of the hippuric acid with the alkaline bases are much more soluble than the corresponding compounds of uric acid, Dr. Ure supposes that the substitution of the former for the latter may be the means of preventing tophaceous concretions, &c. He remarks that, "the application of the above principle has proved of material benefit in the treatment of certain unhealthy conditions of the urine, occurring in subjects of a calculous or gouty diathesis, since it enables the practitioner to obviate entirely the various depositions resulting from the excess of uric acid, the fruitful source of that most distressing malady, stone in the bladder; as also to control and prevent the formation of the so-called tophaceous concretions or chalk stones, which occasion so much inconvenience, deformity and pain to individuals laboring under gout."*

Wilhelm Keller states that, "so early as the edition of Berzelius' 'Lehrbuch der Chemie,' published in 1831, Professor Wöhler had expressed the opinion that benzoic acid, during digestion, was probably converted into hippuric acid." This statement was recalled to mind by the publications of Dr. Ure; and Mr. Keller

*Provincial Med. & Surg. Journal, July 17th, 1841, p. 317.

was induced to experiment upon himself. He took in the evening, before bed-time, about thirty-two grains of pure benzoic acid, in syrup. During the night he perspired strongly, which was probably an effect of the acid, as he was in general with great difficulty made to perspire profusely. He could perceive no other effect, even when, next day, he took the same dose three times; indeed, even the perspiration did not again occur. The urine voided the next morning, when treated with muriatic acid, yielded considerable hippuric acid, but it also contained its normal proportions of urea and uric acid. Keller remarks that, "this observation is opposed to the statement of Dr. Ure, and that he is certainly too hasty in recommending benzoic acid as a remedy for the gouty and calculous concretions of uric acid."

Dr. Walker,* of Huddersfield, England, remarks, that, so far as "he can judge from the exhibition of benzoic acid in several cases of dysuria senilis, he is inclined to augur very favorably of its utility," and that "it is often of service where the gravel in the urine is inconsiderable, and where the irritation and the pain would seem to have arisen from some other cause." He employed it in conjunction with balsam copaiba.

Dr. Soden,† of Bath, England, relates a case of irritability of the bladder, with muco-purulent discharge and enlargement of the prostate, in which he administered the benzoic acid, mixed with balsam copaiba, white of egg and camphor mixture. He says that he "never witnessed any thing equal to the efficacy of this medicine; the urine became clearer after the first dose, and in two days it was perfectly free from mucous deposit; the irritability of the bladder was lessened, and in four days the patient resumed his self-management."

A case in which the urine was loaded with phosphatic salts, treated by Mr. Farquhar, of London, and reported by Dr. Ure, will be found among the cases in the appendix to this article.

* Provincial Med. & Surg. Journal, Feb. 26th, 1842.
† Ibid, July 29th, 1842.

In the following list of symptoms, those which are not accredited to some one else, are such as have been observed by myself, and have been the result of homœopathic attenuations of benzoic acid.

HEAD.—Confusion of the head with drowsiness.

Pain in the temples in the region of constructiveness.

Pressure on the whole of the upper part of the head and spinal column, as if these were pressed together by an elastic body, so that he bends himself involuntarily, stretching forwards. This sensation, without being painful, is productive of extraordinary anxiety. (Occurring two days in succession whilst sitting. Forenoon. *Lingen.*)

Itching of the scalp.

EYES. 5.—Itching in the angles of the eyes.

EARS.—Itching in the left ear.

Shooting pain in the right ear; intermitting.

NOSE.—Sensation of irritation in the left nostril, such as precedes sneezing, yet without being able to sneeze.

Slight transitory hoarseness and repeated sneezing, in the morning, with a pleasant excitement and freedom of the head, which, together with its more rapid disappearance, distinguished it from the ordinary symptoms of taking cold of the experimenter. (7th day, *Lingen.*)

TEETH.—Slight cutting pain in the teeth.

Darting pain in carious molars in both jaws.

LIPS.—Involuntary biting of the lower lip at dinner, on two successive days. (*Lingen.*)

MOUTH.—Soreness of the back part of the tongue, felt most whilst swallowing.

Sensation of soreness and rawness at the root of the tongue, and on the palate.

15. * Extensive ulcerations of the tongue, with deeply chapped or fungoid surfaces.

* An ulcerated tumour in the left side of the mouth,

upon the soft commissure of the jaws behind the last molar teeth.

THROAT.—Heat in the œsophagus, as from acid eructation.

STOMACH.—Singultus.

Sensation of heat throughout the abdomen.

20. Pain in the left side of the abdomen immediately below the short ribs.

BOWELS.—Bowels freely open with extraordinary pressure to stool.

* Fœtid, watery, white stools, very copious and exhausting in infants, the urine being of a very deep red color.

URINE.—Irritability of bladder, too frequent desire to evacuate the bladder, the urine normal in appearance.

Urine at first only increased in quantity and not in frequency. In a few days urination became exceedingly frequent with strong pressing. Urine of an aromatic odor, and saline taste; the odor long retained, most in the forenoon. (*Lingen.*)

25. * Urine highly colored, sometimes of the color of brandy, the urinous odor exceedingly strong.

* Urine of the above character, of a specific gravity greater than that of healthy urine passed into the same vessel, retaining its place below the healthy urine without admixture, and though of a very deep red color, depositing no sediment.

* Hot, scalding urine of a deep red color and strong odor, causing so much suffering in its passage, that this was performed but once a day.

SEXUAL.—A thrilling almost painful sensation on the left side of the glans penis, extending into the urethra, so severe as to occasion starting, ending in a sensation of tickling and itching.

Itching in the sulcus behind the corona glandis.

30. Smarting of the frænum præputii.

LARYNX.—Sneezing, with slight hoarseness, without accompanying catarrhal symptoms. (*Lingen.*)

* Troublesome, and almost constant, dry hacking cough.

CHEST.—Pain about the third rib on the right side, midway between the sternum and the side.

Pain in the right side of the back about midway between the tenth vertebra dorsalis and the side.

35. Pain in the left side about the sixth rib, increased by deep inspiration, and by bending the body to either side.

Deep penetrating pain in the posterior part of the left side, about the sixth rib.

BACK.—Dull pain in the back in the region of the kidneys.

EXTREMITIES.—Knicking and cracking of the joints, both of the superior and inferior extremities, in motion.

Pain in the joints of the fingers of the right hand.

40. The pain leaves the right hand and appears in the left arm, then extends downward into the elbow and leaving this situation next appears in the region of the heart.

The pain having left these parts, appears in the right thigh and ankle.

Pain in the right tendo achilles, and in the region of the heart at the same time.

The pain is incessantly and suddenly changing its location, but its most constant seat is in the region of the heart.

After leaving the right, the pain appears in the left tendo achilles.

45. Aching pain in the left hip, then in the thigh, next in the knees, then in the toes.

Sharp pain in the left ankle, during the time it supports the weight of the body whilst walking.

Upon supporting a slight part of the weight of the body on the left foot, severe pain in the tendo achilles close to the os calcis.

Pain in the gastrocnemii.

Pain in the toes.

50. * Pain in the large joints of the great toes, with slight tumefaction and redness.

Stitch passing perpendicularly upwards, through the right great toe, followed by a burning which increases gradually again to a stitch; appearing afterwards in the left great toe, from which it vanishes with a thrilling sensation, in the morning, whilst lying down. (The 8th day, *Lingen.*)

Itching on various parts of the body and extremities, yielding rather an agreeable feeling on being scratched, but leaving a burning.

Feeling of coldness of the knees as if they were blown upon by a cold wind. (9th day. *Lingen.*)

Frequent pulse. (The 1st, 2nd and 3rd day. *Lingen.*)

SLEEP.—55. Awakened after midnight with violent pulsation of the heart and temporal arteries, (pulsation 110 in the minute,) without external heat; and cannot fall asleep again. In the morning, the tongue covered with a white mucous coat; nausea and total loss of appetite. In the afternoon at 4 o'clock, all these symptoms had vanished. (The 4th day. *Lingen.*)

He awakens every morning about 2 o'clock, from strong internal heat, and a hard, bounding, but not quickened pulse, so that he must lie awake upon his back, because the pulsation of the temporal arteries, sounds like puffing in the ears, and prevents him from going to sleep again. (Enduring for 8 weeks. *Lingen.*)

APPENDIX.

In the introduction to this article, some remarks in relation to certain remedial operations of the benzoic acid, have already been made. But it is necessary to enter more into detail in regard to its therapeutic action.

Evincing, as it does, such decided influence over the

kidneys, it is expected to exert remedial power in many diseases in which the deviations of these organs from the normal performance of their functions constitute an important part of the morbid derangement. This view is not only confirmed by the statements already made, but also by experiences of my own; many of them, long anterior to the earliest of these publications.

I have found the benzoic acid of great utility in a number of cases where the urine was of a deep red colour, sometimes even as dark as brandy, and its urinous odor peculiarly strong.

This highly colored and strongly scented urine, occurs most frequently in syphilitic cases, where the external symptoms have been either wholly or partially suppressed by improper treatment; also in some cases after the infection, but before the establishment of chancre or syphilitic gonorrhœa; and sometimes accompanies these disorders. It is often so strongly marked as to attract the attention of the patient sufficiently to induce him to remark it to the physcian. A few cases in illustration may be useful.

Case.—A lad about seventeen years of age had contracted a chancre, and by the advice of acquaintances, had taken balsam copaiba and other medicines. The chancre disappeared; but was succeeded by the following disease:—Slightly elevated, raw surfaces, of a wart-like appearance, and of a circular form, varying in diameter from half an inch to an inch and a half, at places running into each other; nearly covered both sides and the bottom of the sulcus ani, and caused much smarting and soreness of the part. Thuya and mercury were given without much apparent effect. Benzoic acid, in high dilution, and in a single dose, restored to its normal character, the urine, which was previously very highly colored and strongly scented; and effected some improvement in the disease. When the urine again became highly colored, the dose was repeated, and with such good results, that it was afterwards given every two or three days until the cure was completed.

Case.—I was called to visit a gentleman aged 25 years, whom I found suffering under a tormenting, almost constant, dry, hacking cough. His room-mate had informed me that he suspected him of laboring under syphilitic disease, from the fact that his urine was of the character above described. (My informant was acquainted with the value of the symptom, having been under my care for a syphilitic rheumatism, and experienced much benefit from the use of the benzoic acid.) Upon inquiry, I found that he had, a short time before the commencement of his cough, labored under a gonorrhœa, for the cure of which he had recourse to the ordinary methods of treatment. The benzoic acid speedily restored the urinary secretion to its ordinary quality, and the cough soon ceased to be troublesome.

Case.—A man aged about 23 years, who had a chancre cured a year or two before by external applications, and whose health from that time had not been good, suffered at the time he called upon me, with syphilitic rheumatism. The use of the benzoic acid was followed by the disappearance of the rheumatism and a re-appearance of the chancre. In the treatment of the latter affection I was so far from successful that he applied to another physician, who, by means of external applications, &c. succeeded in removing it, without any very troublesome return of the rheumatism.

Rather seeking to avoid venereal practice, my experience in this direction is not very extensive, especially in the treatment of the recent forms of the disease, yet still it is sufficient, both from the above and other cases, to justify me in recommending the benzoic acid as a remedy worthy of attention in the treatment of syphilis, and more especially in the secondary forms of this disease.

It is not only where the syphilitic taint exists that this remedy proves serviceable, but it is also of great utility in many cases where there cannot be a suspicion entertained of its presence. In several cases of angina faucium and angina tonsillaris, where the urine possessed the characteristics above mentioned, the benzoic acid has proved itself very useful. In two cases, of a mother and her daughter, a young woman, both for a long time subject to violent angina, in neither of whom the allopathic treatment had ever succeeded in preventing suppuration, though early and energetically applied, and where, in the case of the daughter, homœopathic treatment with belladonna and other apparently indicated remedies had twice failed to prevent suppuration, although it diminished the suffering much more than any previous treatment, benzoic acid in alternation with belladonna and digitalis would speedily subdue the attacks, and finally seemed to effect such an alteration of the system that the tendency to this form of disease appeared to be almost extinguished.

Dr. Williamson has communicated to me the case of a man subject to annual returns of nephritic colic, the urine extremely highly colored and strongly scented, where the benzoic acid afforded great relief in a paroxysm two years ago, since which he has not had his usual returns of the complaint.

In cases of diarrhœa in infants, where the stools are very copious, watery, very light colored and fœtid, and where the urine is of an uncommonly deep red color, and its urinous odor remarkably strong, I have found the benzoic acid produce very great improvement.

In the cases where the ulcerations of the tongue described in the list of symptoms occurred, the urine was of the character above described, but there was no reason to suppose syphilitic taint.

The following case is the one mentioned in the introduction as treated by Mr. Farquhar and reported by Dr. Ure:*

"H. H., aged thirty-seven, of spare make and sedentary habits, consulted me on the 9th of May, 1842, relative to a disorder of the urinary secretion. He said that about ten months previously he noticed, for the first time, a whitish deposit in his water, which, ere long, concreted on the chamber-pot, forming

* Provincial Med. and Sur. Journal, Feb. 11, 1843, p. 690.

a hard grey crust, most difficult to remove; the urine had a very offensive odor, and varied occasionally in appearance, presenting sometimes a greenish, at other times a brownish color; at the above date it was slightly opaque and of a pale yellow hue, emitting a pungent ammoniacal smell, alkaline to litmus, and effervescing briskly upon the addition of a few drops of hydrochloric acid; almost as soon as discharged it threw down a white flocculent sediment, consisting of phosphate and carbonate of lime; it did not afford any uric acid; its specific gravity was 1.023; it was voided without pain or difficulty, and in a full stream; there was little or no increase of the mucous secretion, and no albumen. The patient's appetite was good, his tongue clean, and he slept well; but he was pale, complaining of general lassitude and languor, and of a sense of weakness across the loins; his bowels were generally confined. 1000 grains measure of the above urine, evaporated to dryness by a water bath at a temperature not exceeding 160° Fah., left only thirty-six grains of dry extract, and exhaled, during the process a great quantity of ammonia, as proved by a slip of moist litmus paper held over the dish becoming instantaneously blue. He was directed to take an aperient dose of rhubarb and ten grains of benzoic acid, twice in the day, and to live well, but plainly.

May 12. Has taken the medicine without suffering the slightest inconvenience. He says that the urine, within a few hours after the first dose, became clear, and ceased to deposit any chalky sediment. It is now natural in all respects; acid to litmus; specific gravity 1.022. After six days longer he discontinued the use of the benzoic acid. Towards the end of the month the urine became again alkaline, and I was induced to try him with the usual routine of medicines recommended in cases of this description, in order to see whether the urine could be brought to a permanently moral state."

This was done, but without benefit. A renewal of the use of the benzoic acid led to most satisfactory results.

In many cases of rheumatism and of painful joints with arthritic concretions, I have had reason to believe that the benzoic acid has proved of great advantage. Very striking effects may be observed from this remedy in arthritic irritation of the great toe joints, attended with swelling and redness of the skin, the irritation being mostly confined to these parts, and the urine of the character above mentioned. I was yesterday conversing with a patient who was formerly very much troubled with this complaint, to whom I gave the benzoic acid about six years ago, when the disease disappeared in twenty-four hours, and never re-appeared until within a few weeks of the present time, when it again showed itself in a very slight degree.

In a case where inflammatory rheumatism and violent asthma, both of long standing and frequent recurrence, co-existed, and for which I gave the benzoic acid, the patient remarked a great amelioration of his asthmatic paroxysms. This is worthy of mention, inasmuch as one of the benzoated tinctures of opium was formerly termed Elixir asthmaticum, and it may be that further observations will prove the benzoic acid to be a remedy for some peculiar forms of asthmatic disorder.

ACIDUM FLUORICUM.

BY C. HERING, M. D.

Acidum Hydrofluoricum. Fluss-spathsaeure, Germ. Fluoric Acid.

THIS acid was first procured in its pure state in the year 1810, by Gay-Lussac and Thenard. It is prepared by acting on the mineral called fluor spar, carefully separated from silicious earth, and reduced to fine powder, with twice its weight of concentrated sulphuric acid. Most chemists are now in favour of the opinion of Ampère and Davy, namely, that fluor spar is a compound of fluorine and calcium, and that pure hydrofluoric acid evinces no sign of containing either oxygen or water, but is a compound of fluorine and hydrogen.

Hydrofluoric acid is at 32° a colourless fluid, and remains in that state at 59°, if preserved in well stopped bottles; but when exposed to the air, it flies off in dense white fumes, which consist of the acid vapour combined with the moisture of the atmosphere. Its specific gravity is 1.0609, but its density may be increased to 1.25 by gradual additions of water. Its affinity for this liquid far exceeds that of the strongest sulphuric acid, and the combination is accompanied with a hissing noise, as when red-hot iron is quenched by immersion in water.

It has all the characters of a powerful acid. It has a strong sour taste, reddens litmus paper, and neutralizes alkalies, either forming salts termed *hydrofluates*, or most generally giving rise to metallic fluorides. All these compounds are decomposed by strong sulphuric acid, with the aid of heat, and the hydrofluoric acid, while escaping, may be detected by its action on glass. (*Turner.*)

It is a solvent for some elementary principles, which resist the action even of nitro-hydrochloric acid. Thus it dissolves silicon, zirconium, and columbium, with evolution of hydrogen gas; and when mixed with nitric acid, it proves a solvent for silicon, which has been condensed by heat, and for titanium. Nitro-hydrofluoric acid, however, is incapable of dissolving gold and platinum. Several oxidized bodies, which are not attacked by sulphuric, nitric, or hydrochloric acid, are readily dissolved by hydrofluoric acid. As examples of this fact, several of the weaker acids, such as silica or silicic acid, titanic, columbic, molybdic, and tungstic acids may be enumerated. (*Berzelius.*)

Its vapour is much more pungent than chlorine, or any of the irritating gases. Of all substances, it is the most destructive to animal matter. The following quotations from different authors will bear witness of its powerful action on the cuticle:

Of all bodies fluoric acid, perhaps, produces the strongest caustic effects; it acts most powerfully on the animal tissue, on coming in contact with the skin; there ensues a violent pain; the parts around the spot touched by it become white and painful, forming a dense vesicle filled with matter. Even a very small, hardly visible quantity would produce the same effects, although only after several hours. (*Thenard.*)

This acid unites itself with the skin to such a degree, that even by means of carbonate of soda it cannot be washed off, although the pain is mitigated by the application of the latter; it is also relieved by opening the vesicle as speedily as possible; in the case of the diluted or silicious fluoric acid, the presence of water or silicious acid prevents these effects. (*Berzelius.*)

The smallest quantity applied to the hand excites violent itching, and pustules filled with matter are formed. (*Liebig.*)

A solution of one-forty-eighth part of a grain produced on the skin neither pain nor redness, neither did a solution of one-sixteenth. One-eighth of a grain, however, applied to the skin produced some pain, redness, heat; the epidermis came off in scales after a few days. (*Kreiner.*)

Fluoric acid acts energetically on glass. The transparency of the glass is instantly destroyed, heat is evolved and the acid boils, and in a short time entirely disappears. A colourless gas, known by the name of fluo-silicic acid gas is the product. This compound is always formed when hydrofluoric acid comes in contact with a silicious substance. For this reason it cannot be preserved in glass; but must be prepared and kept in metallic vessels. Those of lead, on account of their cheapness, are often used, but silver or platinum are preferable. (*Turner.*)

The following symptoms are the result of the provings of a number of individuals, whose names are appended to each symptom of their proving; where possible, also, the period which elapsed between the taking of the medicine and the time of the appearance of the symptom, has been added. The numbers after the symptoms refer to the degree of the attenuation, taken by the prover. The symptoms without numbers were produced by the thirtieth potence; and those marked with a * are curative.

MENTAL.—*Disposition to anxious ideas*, frequently to such a degree that a perspiration breaks out. (2d day. 3*d*. *Hering*.)

He is less anxious than formerly. (30*th*. *Hering*.)

In the evening he is very discontented; he looks at every thing in the worst light; in the morning, after a restless night, his temper is very cheerful and joyous. (6*th*. *Hering*.)

Easily displeased for half a day. (After 14 hours. 30*th*. *Campos*.)

5. The least trifle is with him sufficient, to show a bad temper in his features and motions in 16 hours; disappears after 12 hours. (*Campos.*)

Ill humour after 18 hours, lasts about 12 hours. (*Campos.*)

Whilst considering what might happen, he gets into a most ungovernable anger, but only in his thoughts. Several times during the first days. (3*d.* *Hering.*)

Great disposition, when alone, to repulsive fantastic imaginations, particularly with regard to persons with whom he stands in near relations, or with whom he is connected. (3*d.* *Hering.*)

* A lame and imbecile old lady dismissed her nurse, without which she could not get along at all, quarrelled with her nieces, could not bear the sight of them, and tormented, without cause, the whole house. After two doses, 30*th*, evening and morning, she had a running from the eyes, and was immediately patient and cheerful, and remained so. (*Hering.*)

10. During the fourth week very irritable towards people, even to the greatest hatred, which he does not hesitate to give vent to in words; but as soon as he sees them every thing is forgotten, and he has an entirely different opinion of them. This does not arise either from hypocrisy or cowardice, but it is a suddenly altered view, mentally the same feeling which occurred to him physically during the coryza, 298, 300. (3*d.* *Hering.*)

Aversion to his business. (12*th.* *Gosewisch.*)

Indifferent, showing no interest in any occupation. (3*d.* *Hering.*)

Perfect *contentment, every thing is right.* (*Campos.*)

Feeling of an interior happy state, never experienced before, next morning after the remedy. (*Campos.*)

Uncommonly gay disposition of the mind, the next morning after taking it. (*Campos.*)

15. All nature around seems to smile, in the morning, 16 hours after taking the remedy. (*Campos.*) Comp. 108.

Feeling of perfect happiness within and without, after 8 hours. (*Campos.*)

Satisfaction, he desires no better state of things, *all is right*; after 16 hours. (*Campos.*)

Feeling of highly enjoying everything; after 12 hours. (*Campos.*)

The fourth and the following days a higher grade of well being; he is more decided in his movements. (30*th. Hering.*)

20. He is more cheerful and vigorous after the eighth and following days. (*Hering.*)

Sensation as if dangers did menace him, but without being afraid; particularly during the pressure in the occiput, during the staggering, the pain in the bladder, etc. (3*d. Hering.*)

During the headache, 75, symptoms of the throat, 189. He remembers his experimentation only with horror and aversion, particularly the disagreeable sensation in the stomach, 204, after several weeks, in one who has made numerous provings. (*Williamson.*)

During the tottering sensation, 134, he has a decided though not anxious expectation, as if there was to happen something awful, but he feels no anxiety. 3*d.* (*Hering.*)

It appears to him in the morning as if his countenance had suddenly become old. (The 9th day. 3*d. Hering.*)

25. Difficulty of recalling thoughts after interruption. (30*th. Hering.*)

A more difficult comprehension of philosophical works; on the other hand all facts appear to be clearer to him. (30*th. Hering.*)

He has great difficulty to fix his attention upon any thing. (12*th. Gosewisch.*)

On making his notes he mistakes right and left, a circumstance that does not easily happen to him. (2d day. 6*th. Hering.*)

Forgetful; he does not recollect sometimes the most common things. (12*th. Gosewisch.*)

30. Forgetfulness of dates and his common employments. (The 2d week. 3*d*. *Hering*.)

HEAD.—Whilst sitting, a frequent sensation of a general shaking, with a dull pressure and compression in the occiput, particularly towards the right; with the continual internal sensation of numbness in the left forearm, and a severe pricking in it whilst stretching it. (The 1st forenoon. 3*d*. *Hering*.)

In the forenoon, after 10 o'clock, a kind of shaking in the head, particularly in the back part of it, and more towards the right; at first whilst sitting, during each quick, short movement, on rising, turning, during walking. (The first week. 3*d*. *Hering*.) Comp. 82.

Vertigo with sickness of stomach. 179.

Slight feeling of nausea and vertigo. 180.

Painful determination of blood to the forehead, like a quick jerk, at the beginning of walking after standing, not after sitting; in the evening three or four hours after taking it. (3*d*. *Hering*.)

It appeared to him to proceed from the throat to the head, he felt as if he was to be struck by apoplexy; a kind of determination of blood to the head and loss of consciousness, he could not recollect where he was. Observed after smelling the acid. (*Hering*.) Comp. 192.

Determination of blood to the head. 79, 42.

From the nape of the neck to the occiput, a feeling like a warm breath. 359.

35. In the morning dulness of the head until breakfast. (From the 3d to the 11th day. 30*th*. *Pehrson*.)

Dulness of the head in the morning, with slight drawing in the right side of the head the 5th and 7th day. (30*th*. *Pehrson*.)

Dulness of the head immediately; sensation as if the brain was pressed upwards. (After 4 weeks. 31*st*. *Geist*.)

Dulness of the occiput only, immediately after repeated doses. (30*th*. *Geist*.)

Dulness towards the right in the occiput after one hour. (3*d*. *Hering*.)

40. Dulness and painful tension in the head towards the right after several hours. (6*th*. *Hering*.)

A stunning sensation in the head, mostly in front, immediately after taking the 5th dilut. (*Williamson.*)

A sensation somewhat resembling numbness or burning, first in the forehead, afterwards in the upper jaw, and lower jaw of the same side, and appearing in the lower part of the occiput and in the bladder, the first evening and next morning. (After taking the 3*d*, and also 6*th* and 30*th* dilution. *Hering*.) Comp. 134, 135.

Confusion and pain through the head after 5 minutes. (*Jeanes.*)

Heaviness of the head; with a dull pain (douleur sourde) deep in the middle of the forehead after two hours. (30*th*. *Campos.*)

45. Five minutes after taking it, there commenced an increase of the flow of saliva, which caused him to spit constantly for about 10 minutes, when he began to feel a pain in the head, a sensation as if the head was too heavy and would drop down from one side to the other, a pressing outward from within; the flow of saliva after this pain had established itself began to diminish, and in about one hour ceased entirely. (2*d*. *E. Smith.*)

A dull heavy pain in the upper part of the forehead; passing sometimes to the upper part of both temples, but more particularly to the left. This pain is increased on stooping; in the evening, one hour and a half after taking it. (1*st*. *E. Smith.*)

The feeling of heaviness in the head continues in a diminished degree until going to bed; he awakes with it in the morning, and it only leaves him at 9 o'clock, A. M. (2*d*. *E. Smith.*)

Heaviness above the eyes; with nausea; worse on motion after 2 and 3 hours. (2*d*. *Neidhard.*)

Soon after taking the medicine, there commenced the same salivation, with a dull heaviness and pain in the whole head. (1*st*. *E. Smith.*)

50. Headache from the nape of the neck upwards, a dull pressure; it appears to proceed from the

nape of the neck through the centre of the head towards the forehead; it concentrates gradually more towards the left as if a throbbing was to arise there. 2 hours after the 5th dose. (*Geist.*) Compare 333, 334, 335.

Pressing pains in the forehead, as if it were in the bone, at the same time also in the bones of the temples; on lying down she feels it all over, but it soon passes away. (Afternoon. B.)

Dull heavy pain in the forehead. (*Esrey.*)

Compressing pain in the right frontal protuberance. (15 minutes after. 2*d.* *Williamson.*)

54. Pressing pain in the forehead, on stooping, also pressing on the right eye. (The 3d day. *Husmann.*)

Painful tension in the head towards the right. 40.

He awakes in the morning with a slight pain in the forehead, which soon passes away. After taking it in the evening. (1*st.* *E. Smith.*)

A pain of short duration in the right side of the forehead the next forenoon. (*Husmann.*)

Headache in the upper part of forehead and vertex towards the right. (After 5 minutes. 3*d.* *Hering.*)

In the evening, after lying down, pain in the forehead and eye towards the right. (The 2d day. *Husmann.*)

Pain in the right frontal protuberance in the evening. (The 4th day. 2*d.* *Williamson.*)

60. Headache in the left side of the forehead, in the evening. (2*d.* *Neidhard.*)

Headache in forehead and temples. (6*th.* *Freitag.*)

Immediately in both temples a severe pressing from within outward for half an hour, after that a pinching pain in the left deltoid muscle. (*Geist.*)

Pressure in both temples, quarter of an hour after the fifth dose. (*Geist.*)

In both temples pressure towards the exterior after one hour. (*Geist.*)

65. Pain in the left temple proceeding from within. (*Freitag.*)

Headache, pressive in both temples after 4 hours. (2*d.* *Neidhard.*)

In the forehead, in the room and open air, a headache, a kind of fulness in the left parietal bone on a spot which he cannot designate very clearly. (The 8th and 9th day. 3*d*. *Hering*.)

Heavy pain in the left half of the head in the course of the coronal suture. (The next morning. 2*d*. *Williamson*.)

In the evening, after an animated conversation, heat in the face and headache, like a pressing and forcing deep interiorly towards the left; appearing at times and subsiding again; it then passes to the left upper jaw, as if the teeth ached, even on those places where the roots of the teeth had been extracted a year ago. (The 2d day. 6*th*. *Hering*.)

70. Suddenly a severely pressing pain on the left side of the occiput; disappears as quickly, but soon returns again. (After one hour. *Geist*.)

Dull pressure in the occiput towards the right. 31.

Pressure in both sides of the occiput beneath the protuberances. (After one hour. *Geist*.)

In the morning shortly after awakening, a cramp-like pain in the very lowest part of the occiput towards the left. (*Husmann*.)

Severe pressure in the left temple. (After 2 hours. *Geist*.)

Pressing pain in the left temple. 425.

Sharp darting pain, from near the posterior superior angle of the right parietal bone to the mastoid process of the right temporal bone; the pain was different from any other; much worse than a prolonged electrical shock or compression of the ulnar nerve. (After 3 days. *Campos*.)

75. Sharp, shooting, undulating pain; it arises on the left side about the middle and near the sutura interparietalis, and proceeds with the quickness of lightning to the left temple near the exterior part of the orbital cavity. This pain shoots for about two seconds, but the undulation lasts a little longer, and it is only when the undulation is nearly over that the mind takes cog-

nizance of the whole of it; the shooting, *and* painful undulation, and the quickness, are of such a nature, that produce immediately in the mind a very disagreeable idea of some impending danger. The undulation may be better compared to that of the streak left on a wall, in darkness, by the friction of a phosphoric match. (*Campos.*)

Shooting pain in the left side of the forehead. (2*d.* *Esrey.*)

Violent jerking in the interior behind and above the right eye-brow, in the bone. (After one hour. 3*d.* *Hering.*) Comp. 449.

On bending the head, as in the act of stooping, a dull, quick, throbbing pain in the right temple, lasting only for a short time. (Evening 8½ o'clock. 2*d.* *E. Smith.*)

A few minutes, after taking the remedy, determination of blood to the head, with heat in forehead, gradually increasing to a headache in os frontis. (2*d.* *Neidhard.*)

80. Pain over the right eyebrow, which disappears, but a similar pain appears for a short time in the right small toe. (The next forenoon. *Husmann.*)

A pain, at first like a contraction on top of the head towards the right, and afterwards under the right shoulder blade. (The next forenoon. *Husmann.*) Compare 36, 112.

After breakfast the pains cease, except in the head, on quickly moving it from one position to the other, which continues the whole day. (The 2d day. 1*st.* *E. Smith.*)

Singular indescribable weakness, like a numbness, as if she had received an electric shock, particularly in the head and in the hands, with nausea in stomach, without desire to vomit. She never experienced a similar sensation. A few days previously she had taken acid. nitr., after that fluor. ac. (30*th.* *Hering.*) Comp. 179, 180, 48.

Itching on the head, which causes him to scratch. (After one hour. 30*th*. *Geist.*)

85. The 9th day, for the first time, desires to scratch the head, without, however, any feeling of itching, and the next morning a very geat falling off of the hair. (3*d*. *Hcring.*)

* He had been becoming more and more bald for two years; about two months after taking the acid a new growth of hair was discovered, which continued to grow, and he is now much less bald than before. (*Williamson.*)

EYES.—Drawing around the right eye. (In the evening after 15 minutes. 2*d*. *Williamson.*) Comp. 80.

Elevated red blotches over the eye brows, most abundant on the left side, but of longer continuance on the right. (The 3d and the following day. 2*d*. *Williamson.*)

Scaly eruption, with pricking sensation in the eyebrows. (The 3d day. 2*d*. *Williamson.*)

90. Burning itching in the right eyebrow, disappears after scratching. (1st hour after 5th dose. *Geist.*) Comp. 101.

Itching, inducing him to scratch on both upper eyelids. (The 1st evening. 3*d*. *Hering.*)

A violent itching at the left inner canthus of the eye, which causes him to scratch very quickly and forcibly. (The 12th day. 3*d*. *Hering.*)

In the evening itching in the right internal canthus of the eye. (2*d*. *Neidhard.*)

Pricking and burning in the internal canthus of the eye. (Evening 2d day. 30*th*. *Husmann.*)

95. Has often an itching in the eyes, which makes him scratch. (1st week. 3*d*. *Hering.*)

Painful itching in the left eye, as if from a grain of sand. (*Esrey.*)

Quivering above the external canthus of the left eye, in one who never had the like. (2d day. 30*th*. *Hering.*)

Quivering externally on the right eye, and soon after a pain similar to that described, 411 and 412, at the bottom of the orbital cavity, after several hours. (30*th*. *Hering.*)

The eye remains affected for several days, so that he has to wink and rub it. (*Hering.*)

100. The vapour of it affects the eye very much. *Liebig.*

Itching burning on a small spot near the right eye externally. (After several hours. *Hering.*)

Burning in the eyes in 15 minutes. (2*d*. *Neidhard.*)

Increased lachrymation. (2*d*. *Esrey.*)

Slight fever heat under the eyes soon after the 2d dose. (1*st*. *E. Smith.*)

105. Pressure as it were behind the right eyeball. (The 2d hour. *Geist.*) Comp. 98, 54, 58, 133.

Sensation as if the eyelids were opened by force and a fresh wind was blowing on them; after that, sensation like sand in the eyeball, which had the same feeling as if the eyes were inflamed. (*Campos.*)

* *Clearness of sight*, with increased power of vision; he can read now distinctly small print, that every night previously seemed confused. (*Campos.*)

Pleasant sensation; as if the eyelids were wider opened, or the eyes more prominent, whereby the circle of the vision becomes more enlarged; *the sight clearer*, and he feels a kind of luxurious enjoyment, while looking at the same things he is used to see every day. (*Campos.*) Comp. 15, 187.

On closing the eyes firmly he observes a large bright ring, which quickly vanishes. (In the evening of the 5th day. 3*d*. *Hering.*)

110. In the evening after retiring a jerking light before the eyes, crossing itself like lightning. (The 3d week. 3*d*. *Hering.*)

In the evening after retiring, on closing the eyes, red sparklings cross each other in all possible directions; this gradually ceases, and there remains a red, flaming, trembling for a few minutes, which disappears after opening the eyes. (The 2d day. 1*st*. *Husmann.*)

* A dark spot, which, whilst reading, floats before

his eyes, since he had a violent intermittent fever six years ago, disappeared during the first hour, but returned again in 14 days. (*Geist.*)

EARS. Behind the right ear a pain which moves upwards in the head; at the same time in the right heel. (6*th.* *Freitag.*)

Jerking behind the left ear. (2*d.* *Neidhard.*) Comp. 449.

A peculiar pressing and itching deep in the left ear; disappears after stirring with the finger in the ear. (After one hour. *Geist.*)

115. Itching first in the right ear, afterwards in the left ear. (*Geist.*)

Pressing pain in the right ear. (*Husmann.*)

Pain in the right ear the 4th day. (6*th.* *Freitag.*)

Stitches in the right ear. (30*th.* *Freitag.*)

Sensation in the right ear as if there would commence a ringing in the ear. (In the forenoon the 2d day. 3*d.* *Hering.*)

120. The sensitiveness of his hearing is very much increased in the morning. (The 6th day. 3*d.* *Hering.*)

NOSE. * A chronic inflammation of the nose with pain; redness, some swelling and heat, (on the right interior side of the tip, and in the base of the right wing) disappears within 3 days; there forms itself on the latter place a small pustule, with even surface, on a painful red circle. (6*th.* *Hering.*)

The nose, which for many months was free from excoriation or pain, begins again to feel sore, and more towards the left. (The 9th day. 3*d.* *Hering.*)

In the morning there appears a pimple of the size of a hempseed, towards the right, between the root of the nose and the eye. The 16th day. Several similar pimples in the right side of the face after 5 weeks. (3*d.* *Hering.*)

* A pimple with inflamed base very extensive on the top of the nose, three-quarters of an inch from the tip. (Cured in 2 days. 15*th.* *Jeanes.*)

FACE AND JAWS. 125. Heat in the face, and

desire to bathe the face with cold water, and repeated ablutions, which he much enjoys; for two weeks, after that less decidedly. (*3d. Hering.*) Comp. 69, 74, 104.

Perspiration particularly in the face. (The 3d and the following day. *3d. Hering.*)

Slight itching like fine prickings, on the right side of the face. (After one hour. *Geist.*

Itching on the right side of the face. (*30th. Husmann.*)

Compression in both zygomas, drawing downwards towards the larynx, where she is conscious of it during deglutition, and also without. (In the evening, 5 o'clock. B.) Comp. 457, 5.

130. Deep in the bones, superior and posterior to the left eye, a soreness occasionally. (Evening the 9th day. *3d. Hering.*) Comp. 98.

Behind the left eye towards the temple, in the left nostril and forehead there is a pain, which seems to be in the bone, as if very deeply in the interior something sharp pointed was moved about. (One o'clock in the afternoon the 9th day. *3d. Hering.*)

* The same pain as above described in the case of a fistula lachrymalis of the left eye, with white oblong little scabs and periodical itching every couple of days for several days, and with discharge; fl. ac. *30th* caused the pain immediately to return, but after that every thing was cured. (*Hering.*)

A pain very deep in the posterior part of the right eye, and extending very far into the upper jaw, the same which he had at one o'clock in the left side.) (At 5 and 6 o'clock in the evening, the 9th day. *3d. Hering.*)

Sensation of warmth and obtusion in the bone of the right upper jaw. (After 10 minutes. *3d. Hering.*)

135. Painful sensibility of the right upper jaw. This sensibility is, as it were, reflected in the lower jaw. (After 15 minutes. *3d. Hering.*)

In the right articulation of the jaw sensation as if a spasm were to take place. (After several hours. *Geist.*)

In both joints of the jaws, (worse in the left,) a painful spasmodic contraction. Had the same sensation occasionally before. (The 11th day. 3*d*. *Hering*.)

Slight numbness of the right joint of the lower jaw, a continual sensation of warmth. (After 1 and 2 hours. 3*d*. *Hering*.)

Drawing pain in the right lower jaw bone, towards the middle. (1 hour after the 5th dose. *Geist*.)

140. Slight gnawing pain in both sides of the lower jaw, in the bone near the angle. (Soon after 79. 2*d*. *Neidhard*.)

In connection with a drawing in the entire left eye, a peculiar sensation in the right lower jaw, not in the bone, but very close to it. In the evening, 24 hours after taking the remedy. (30*th*. *Freitag*.) Comp. 454.

Burning pain on the outside of the right lower jaws on a small spot near the first or second molar tooth. (After 1 and 2 hours. 3*d*. *Hering*.)

TEETH.—*Teeth feel warm;* those of the upper jaw especially on the left side. The incisor and canine are much warmer than any of the others. A few minutes afterwards there was considerable warmth in the pharynx. These sensations ceased in the course of an hour. The prover remarked, particularly, that the heat or warmth was felt in the teeth, and not gums or alveolar process. (1*st*. *E. Smith*.)

Digging pain in one of the lower incisors, towards the right. (The 3d day. *Husmann*.)

145. Toothache; drawing in the left lower jaw. (After 4 hours. 2*d*. *Neidhard*.)

Toothache for a short time in the left lower jaw. (30*th*. *Freitag*.)

The right upper incisors are very sensitive on drinking cold water, and also on inhaling cold air, particularly the one which is decayed. (The same symptom some weeks before the proving. 30*th*. *Hering*.) Comp. 159.

The cold air in a room causes pain in the carious tooth of the right upper incisor. (Evening, after several hours. 6*th*. *Hering*.)

Soon after taking the remedy transient pain in the right eye tooth. (Evening. *Husmann.*)

150. The pain in the tooth on the right side disappears for a moment, and is transmitted to the left thigh, on the outside above the knee. (The 3d day. *Husmann.*)

The right eyetooth, which was formerly rough, but became afterwards smooth again, is now rough, and commences to ache, particularly at the root of it. In the upper jaw, along the root of the teeth pressure is very painful, particularly in the evening ; it is mitigated temporarily, by cold water. (The 3d and following days. *Husmann.*)

* A fistula of several years standing near the right eyetooth, with great sensitiveness in touching the upper jaw ; gradually disappears during the provings. (*Hering.*)

The 5th day in the morning the lower incisor teeth have a sensation of roughness, as if they were broken, and the tongue feels painful on touching them. (For several days. *3d. Hering.*)

Acrid putrid taste from the root of the right lateral incisor, on which there is fixed an artificial tooth. (The next morning after. *2d. Williamson.*)

155. * After the second week a decidedly improved condition of his teeth ; the carious teeth seem to secrete less, and the gums do not bleed so easily. (*3d. Hering.*) Comp. 182.

(After five weeks a painful excoriation near the first lower molar tooth, on the right side. *3d. Hering.*)

MOUTH, TASTE, NAUSEA.—A sensation of warmth on the lips. (Immediately. *3d. Hering.*)

Very often a burning, like a sore on the inside of the lower lip towards the right, very near the edge. (After 1 and 2 hours. *3d. Hering.*)

A solution of $\frac{1}{8}$ caused in the mouth a violent pain, as from hot water ; the teeth became so painful that for two days he could not masticate with them *Kreiner.*

160. One drop of the one-sixteenth solution produced in the mouth a bluntness of the teeth, a sensation of sticking, contraction and tension, after which the interior cuticle of the mouth became whitish and peeled off. After three days. *Kreiner.*

Twenty drops of the one-forty-eighth solution, taken in water, excited frequent sour eructations; sensation of heat and a disagreeable flat taste in the mouth. *Kreiner.*

One drop of the one-forty-eighth solution produced in the mouth contractions and prickling, and a disagreeable taste. *Kreiner.*

The taste is quite intolerable. *Thenard.*

In the evening, taste like ink; seems to proceed from a lower tooth on the left side. (2d day. 6*th. Hering.*)

Acrid foul taste from the root of the tooth. 154.

165. In the morning on awakening, a saltish taste in the mouth until breakfast. (The 2d day. *Pehrson.*)

After-taste in the mouth of what he has eaten; worse in the afternoon. (12*th. Gosewisch.*)

Acid taste, and greasy feeling in the mouth immediately after. (3*d. Jeanes.*)

Greasy feeling in the mouth, immediately. (3*d. Hering.*)

Sweetish taste in the throat at night. (4th day. 2*d. Williamson.*)

170. After dinner sour bitter eructations. (In three hours. 2*d. Neidhard.*)

Sour eructations. 161.

Frequent acid eructations, with pyrosis and passage of flatulency. (In the afternoon, the 2d day. 2*d. Neidhard.*)

Eructations with choking. 190.

Frequent nauseating eructations, with inclination to vomit. 202.

Pyrosis with nausea. (In 2½ hours. 2*d. Neidhard.*)

Eructation of wind and sickness of the stomach, very soon. (2*d. Neidhard.*)

Eructation and *discharge of flatulency, frequently.* (*Campos.*)

175. Sickness of stomach, continuing from three to four hours, after taking the acid. (1*st.* *Esrey.*)

Sickness of the stomach with some desire to vomit. (1*st.* *E. Smith.*)

Some sickness of the stomach. (After 4 hours. 2*d.* *Neidhard.*)

Constant great *sickness* of the stomach, with *general heat.* (After 2 hours. 2*d.* *Neidhard.*) Comp. 48, 83.

Continual sickness of stomach, with vertigo and headache. (After 4 hours. 2*d.* *Neidhard.*)

180. Slight feeling of nausea and vertigo. (After 10 minutes. 3*d.* *Hering.*)

He vomits several times with difficulty a clear, viscid fluid, with coagulated white pieces, having no connection with the burning in the mouth, nor the symptoms accompanying it. The whole day he felt *nausea, eructations* and *lassitude.* After 30 drops of one-sixteenth solution, (about 2 grains.) *Kreiner.*

* The mouth is not so full of mucus in the morning as usual; it is less around the teeth; in rincing it there is less blood and viscid mucus than usual. (After several days. 30*th.* *Hering.*)

Five minutes after taking, an increase of the flow of saliva, so that he had to spit constantly for about 10 minutes; after which he began to feel a pain in the head, when the flow of saliva diminished and ceased in one hour. 45, 49.

Much viscid saliva in awakening at night, before the diarrhœa. 231.

Increase of saliva with sneezing. 297.

PALATE AND FAUCES. Prickling of the tongue, and increase of saliva for some hours, and afterwards combined with smarting, feeling of the palate as if something very acrid had been gargled. A feeling of tenderness and irritability in the larynx; coughing to clear the throat causes feeling of soreness, which shows an unusual degree of sensibility. (3*d.* *Jeanes.*) Comp. 162.

* A very painful little ulcer in the lower part of the mouth, towards the right, in the corner of the upper and

lower jaw; very troublesome during mastication and otherwise. (*Hering.*)

185. Sensation of heat in the fauces. (The next morning. *Husmann.*)

Dryness of the left half of the palate and roof of the mouth. (In the evening the 4th day. 2*d.* *Williamson.*)

A singular sensation of expansion in the posterior nares, during his walk in the open air. (30*th.* *Hering.*) Compare eyes, 108.

* A pain to which he was frequently subject at the opening of the left eustachian tube, appears after one to two hours, and does not recur again afterwards. (3*d.* *Hering.*)

In the lower part of the entrance of the fauces, towards the left side a raw feeling; although it is little painful, he still apprehends it may prove serious. (The 11th and 12th day, in the morning and forenoon. 3*d.* *Hering.*)

190. Violent burning in the fauces, and a sensation of constriction; rumbling in the bowels, pressure in the stomach, and burning eructations; choking for two hours; the second day constipated. From 10 drops of the one-sixteenth solution, (about $\frac{5}{8}$ gr.) *Kreiner.*

Immediately a slight itching sensation in the larynx, which causes him to swallow and to hawk, lasting for hours. 2 drops. (31*st.* *Geist.*)

Sore throat, with difficult deglutition; his throat, as far as below the larynx, felt so sore that the bread, although masticated very thoroughly, could not be swallowed without the greatest pain. After the smelling of the acid, 5 o'clock, P. M., until the next morning after breakfast. The same morning hawking up of much phlegm, mixed with some blood; during the day abatement of the symptoms. (*Hering.*)

Constriction in the throat with difficult deglutition, at first in the forenoon, three hours after taking it; the next day it begins towards evening. (30*th.* *Freitag.*)

APPETITE.—With his usual good appetite, he

nevertheless is soon satisfied. (The 3d and 4th day and following days. 30*th*. *Hering*.)

(The same symptom after. 3*d*. *Hering*.)

195. Thirst at night. (*Campos*.)

Appetite increased. (*Campos*.)

Hunger increased. (*Campos*.)

Excessive hunger. (*Campos*.)

Voracious appetite. (*Campos*.) Comp. 222, 250.

200. The appetite is diminished, he wants something "piquant." (12*th*. *Gosewisch*.)

Aversion to coffee the 15th day. (3*d*. *Hering*.)

STOMACH.—Constriction in the throat; pressure and sensation of fulness in the region of the stomach; frequent stale disgusting eructations, with inclination to vomit. Of one drachm of the one-forty-eighth solution, (about one and one-fourth gr.,) within half an hour, all symptoms disappeared. *Kreiner*.

Pressure in the stomach and burning. 190.

Decidedly uncomfortable sensation in the stomach, A. M. (After the 2d dose. 2*d*. *Williamson*.)

Sensitiveness of the region of the stomach to pressure. (12*th*. *Gosewisch*.)

205. Sensation, between meals, as pressure from a weight in the stomach, simulating indigestion. (After 3 days. *Campos*.)

Heat in the stomach before his meal, which disappears after it; then heaviness in the stomach, and after some hours again heat. Worse during exercise. (12. *Gosewisch*.) Comp. 190.

ABDOMEN.—Sensation in the left side of abdomen, as if a pain were to arise and wind discharge, without either taking place. (In half an hour after the fifth dose. *Geist*.) Comp. 228, 231.

Pain in the left side of the abdomen, in the region of the spleen. (After 1 hour. *Geist*.)

Suddenly an acute pain in the left side of abdomen, above the hip, hindering respiration. (After 2 hours. *Geist*.)

210. Pinching in the region of the spleen, forenoon 11 o'clock. (The 4th and following day. *Pehrson*.)

In the evening a pressing pain in the abdomen on the left side, and also in the left arm. (*Freitag.*)

* A pain which he has had for six days in the region of the spleen, reaching to the hips, disappears immediately after one drop 30*th;* and did not return. (*Geist.*)

Jerkings in left side of abdomen. (After 2 hours. *Geist.*)

Pinching in region of navel, excitement to diarrhœa, and a copious watery evacuation. (2 o'clock, A. M. 7th day. *Pehrson.*)

215. During diarrhœa, pain more particularly in region of navel. (Several hours after. 6*th.* *Hering.*)

Immediately after partaking of some pieces of watermelon, a meal of fish, etc., some pain in the abdomen, which is not generally the case. (After 1 hour. 3*d.* *Hering.*)

Rumbling in bowels, with erratic pain. A. M. (1*st.* *E. Smith.*)

Shooting pain in bowels, like as if from wind, sometimes very acute. (Evening. 1*st.* *E. Smith.*)

In the night a sensation of warmth in the abdomen, with a pressure towards the bladder. (1st day. 3*d.* *Hering.*)

220. Throbbing like a pulsation on feeling the breast and abdomen. (B.)

Sensation of faintness, like an emptiness in the region of the navel, with a desire to draw a deep breath. It is relieved by bandaging; in the forenoon, before he had eaten anything; it gets better after eating. In the evening it is more like a slight burning. When occupied he does not observe it. (12*th.* *Gosewisch.*)

Inclination tô draw up the muscles of the abdomen, with great appetite. (12*th.* *Gosewisch.*)

FÆCES.—Free evacuation of the bowels, twice a day. (2*d.* *Williamson.*)

Inclination to diarrhœa; two passages the first day. (2*d.* *Neidhard.*)

225. Two hard passages the 2d day. (2*d.* *Neidhard.*)

Hasty pressure for a passage like in diarrhœa, and a soft evacuation, P. M., 2 o'clock. Three hours after the 4th dose, 30*th*, 4 drops. Was formerly very regular in his bowels. (*Geist.*)

In the evening, ineffectual desire for a passage. (The 5th day. *Pehrson.*)

After eating, rumbling in the stomach, and urging like in diarrhœa. (The 13th and 14th day. *Pehrson.*)

* The soft small passage, which he has every morning after drinking coffee, and again late in the evening, with ineffectual urging and protrusion of hemorrhoids, changes after 4 to 5 days into copious natural evacuations. (30*th. Hering.*)

230. His passage is more loose than common. (12*th. Gosewisch.*)

He wakes up after midnight with a large quantity of viscid, tasteless saliva in the mouth, burning pinching pain in the stomach, and with a sensation of distension from flatulency; after the passage of some wind the pain is increased, and he cannot pass any more; after a copious pappy evacuation of the bowels the pains seem to concentrate themselves in the region of the navel. After the evacuation the pain is diminished; on returning to his room, however, it returns again, and he has a second passage, accompanied with pain in region of the navel; in the morning, 7 o'clock, a third passage. (The 3d day. *Pehrson.*)

4 o'clock, A. M., the same diarrhœa. (6th day. *Pehrson.*)

After rising, a copious pappy evacuation. (The 8th day. *Pehrson.*)

Several pappy evacuations during the 10th day. (*Pehrson.*)

235. Immediately after rising in the morning, two watery stools. (The 12th day. *Pehrson.*) (The passages seem to occur every other day, and every day at a later hour. *Hering.*)

In the morning after rising a pappy loose passage,

the 13th and 14th day; not the 15th; and the 16th, twice, the 17th again once. (*Pehrson.*)

The evacuation becomes protracted, insufficient, and lumpy. (6*th*, 12*th*, 30*th*. *Hering.*)

Passage protracted and very small; the day after, 226, on omitting the remedy. (*Geist.*)

Constipated for two days. After 10 drops one-sixteenth. *Kreiner.*

240. He feels as if the wind was retained in the anus. (6*th*. *Hering.*)

Much rumbling from flatulency. (The 9th day. *Pehrson.*)

Passes much inodorous wind. (12*th*. *Gosewisch.*)

He passes more inodorous flatus, with much noise. (6*th*, 30*th*. After several days. *Hering.*)

Much rumbling in abdomen, 190, 217, 228.

Frequent passage of flatus and eructations; *it leaves him immediately more comfortable, and with a feeling as if that was the last, but is not so; because in a few minutes every thing is renewed in the same order, succession and feeling as before; and so on for two or three days, with the only difference of being at longer intervals than it was at first.* (*Campos.*)

245. In the morning offensive flatus. (The 2d day. *Pehrson.*)

Small very strongly offensive winds precede the evacuation. (2d day. 3*d*. *Hering.*)

The same the 8th day.

Small, excessively offensive discharges of wind in the forenoon, several hours before his meal, and in the afternoon two hours after eating. (The 2d day. 3*d*. *Hering.*)

A large pappy yellowish-brown passage, of a very strong, disagreeable smell of fæces, together with tenesmus to which the prover is liable, although less protrusion of the anus than formerly. (The 2d day. *Hering.*)

The 3d day no passage; the 4th, 10 o'clock, A. M.,

indefinite desire, small odourless winds and pappy evacuation. (*3d. Hering.*)

250. The 8th day, before dinner, after small, excessively fetid discharges of flatus, a sudden urging, then a thin pappy passage without any odour, and at the same time a very copious discharge of urine. He had eaten peaches before, which, however, never acted that way; and after the passage a better appetite than usual. (*3d. Hering.*)

He observed the same tertian type the 2d, 4th, (6th,) and 8th day. (*Hering.*)

The fifth week the evacuation is more regular than usual. (*3d. Hering.*)

ANUS.—Constriction of the anus, in attempting to propel wind. (*6th. Hering.*) Comp. 231, 240.

* The protrusion of the anus during evacuation, habitual to him was very quickly, and to a considerable degree, diminished for several weeks. (*3d. Hering.*)

255. * A more comfortable feeling in the anus than is usual with him; in one subject to piles. (2d day. *3d. Hering.*)

After drinking wine, determination of blood to the anus. (*3d. Hering.*)

Within and around the anus violent itching the 15th and 16th day; continues around the anus until the 5th week. (*3d. Hering.*)

Itching above the anus, suddenly and most violent, often returning. (The 12th and following days. *3d. Hering.*)

Violent itching, which distresses him particularly in the evening, on a small spot in the centre of the perineum. (From the 2d week, increasing until the 6th and 7th. *3d. Hering.*)

GROINS, BLADDER AND URINE.—260. Continual dull pain in the inguinal region on both sides, and deeply situated. (*Campos.*)

Burning for a short time in the right inguinal region. (In the afternoon. *Husmann.*)

Drawing through the left testicle to the abdominal ring. 281.

Dull pains in the region of the bladder. (The 1st week. 3*d*. *Hering*.)

Pressure on the bladder, with a sensation of warmth in the abdomen. 219.

Violent pain like an electric shock from the region of the bladder, down into the right thigh. 411.

Before and after urination, a pain in the lower part of the bladder; there is also pain on pressure. (The 1st and 2d day. 6*th*. *Hering*.)

After urination a pain as it were above the neck of the bladder. (Afternoon. 6*th*. *Hering*.)

265. The frequently returning pain in the bladder is entirely gone. (The 2d day after taking 30*th*. *Hering*.)

In the morning an intolerable burning in the urethra, during urination, and after it for 5 minutes. The 9th day. In one who never had a gonorrhœa. (*Pehrson*.)

Less urination the next morning. (3*d*. *Hering*.)

Decidedly less voiding of urine, the 2d and 3d day, but the urine is not of a darker colour. (3*d*. *Hering*.)

Has to get twice up at night to void his urine, which is quite unusual with him; the night is cooler than the previous ones. (The 5th day. 3*d* *Hering*.)

270. More urination and afterwards more thirst. (The 5th day. 3*d*. *Hering*.)

Urination more frequent, and of a clear colour after several days. (6*th*. *Hering*.)

Frequent desire to make water after several days. (30*th*. *Hering*.)

Free discharge of light coloured urine; very frequent, of sufficiently large, but not increased quantity, leaving him more comfortable; he drinks little as usual. (*Campos*.)

Pungent and strong odour of the urine, which was freely discharged, in the evening. (The 4th day. 2*d*. *Williamson*.)

275. The 15th and 16th day, a very acrid and strong odour of the urine. (3*d*. *Hering*.)

As far as the 6th week, his urine frequently smells very offensively. (3*d*. *Hering*.)

The urine has diminished in quantity and has a decided fragrancy, (like benzoic acid.) (The 2d day, evening and morning. 30*th*. *Hering*.)

His habitual whitish sediment in the urine is also mixed with a very copious purple coloured one. (The 3d day. *Hering*.)

The 5th day his urine has lost its purple coloured sediment and fragrancy. (30*th*. *Hering*.)

280. GENITAL ORGANS.—Sensation of fulness in both spermatic chords. (The 1st evening. 3*d*. *Hering*.) Comp. 260.

Occasionally stiches and drawing through the left testicle, to the abdominal ring and spermatic chord. (After 4 hours. 2*d*. *Neidhard*.)

Sexual passion more easily controlled. (1st week. 3*d*. *Hering*.)

The 6th, 7th and the following days, it seemed as if his sexual desire was disappearing. (For several weeks. 3*d*. *Hering*.)

The 11th morning. The first erections again of very long duration, and quite healthy nature. (3*d*. *Hering*.)

285. An increase of sexual desire the 3d and 4th day, with a complete erection; which, however, soon disappeared. (30*th*. *Hering*.)

Sexual desire increased during the action of fluoric acid. (12*th*. *Gosewisch*.)

Almost irresistible attacks of libidinousness, more in the case of old than young men. (30*th*. *Hering*.)

Sexual passion strong, with violent erections all night, and desire to cohabit. (*Campos*.)

Erections with desire and voluptuousness. (*Campos*.)

290. *Sexual passion increased, with erections at night during sleep.* (*Campos*.)

Highly excessive enjoyment and pleasure during coition, which was not the case before. (*Campos*.)

Seminal discharge not so quick and early as usual, but free and without any bad after feeling. (*Campos*.)

Elderly persons had often attacks of venereal desire and erections, and the exercise of this function seemed not to be injurious to them. (*Hering.*)

The monthly period occurred 8 days too soon, and was more copious; but, instead of 6 to 7 days, lasted only five; the discharge is thick and coagulated. The succeeding catamenia take place again at the regular period, according to the former calculation. (B.)

NOSE, CORYZA.—295. The odour of the acid is very acrid and penetrating. *Thenard.*

Sneezing in the afternoon. (After 4 hours. 2*d. Neidhard.*)

In the morning violent sneezing seven times, with a discharge of a small quantity of thin mucus from the nose, and collection of saliva in the mouth, with that sensation in the nose which arises sometimes from the influence of severely cold weather. (The 2d day. 6*th. Hering.*)

Early in the morning on rincing the mouth with cold water, the nose appears suddenly full of mucus, like as if he had fluent coryza, but as quickly passes over again. (30*th. Hering.*)

Coryza the 8th day, is the 9th day on the right side, and fluent with sneezing; remains semilateral and fluent during the 10th and 11th day. (*Pehrson.*)

* In a case of chronic obstruction of the nose, with a dull heavy pain in the forehead, where silex, 30*th*, had been of some service, fluor. ac. 30*th*, immediately caused a running from the nose, without any other improvement. (The same in a case of ulceration.) (*Husman.*)

300. Sudden attacks of coryza, suddenly appearing and disappearing again; it seems as if excitement removed the coryza. (3*d. Hering.*)

CHEST.—Increased irritability of the larynx; whilst coughing slightly, there arises a sensation of soreness. (*Jeanes.*)

Pain in the larynx as if it were in the cartilage, inducing him to swallow. (After 90 minutes. 3*d. Hering.*)

Soreness in the chest. (After three hours. 2*d*. *Neidhard.*)

A sore pain in the left side of the chest, as if beneath the skin, which he feels only on moving; a similar pain in the left shoulder. (10 o'clock in the evening, after four hours. 1*st*. *E. Smith.*)

305. On rising in the morning, pain again in the left side of the chest, similar to the one he felt the evening before. (1*st*. *E. Smith.*)

Oppression with pain in the chest. (After 4 hours. 2*d*. *Neidhard.*)

Pressing pain in the last rib, towards the right near the spine. (After 1 hour. *Geist.*)

Pressure in the centre of the sternum in the afternoon; in the evening at 10 o'clock after retiring, a pressing pain in the middle of the chest, which lasts until he falls asleep. (The 1st day. *Geist.*)

Small stiches in the side. (After 4 hours. 2*d*. *Neidhard.*)

310. Sticking under the ribs to the left of the ensiform cartilage, in the evening. (After 15 minutes. 2*d*. *Williamson.*)

Burning sticking pain in the left side of the chest, lasting only for a moment. After smelling the acid. (*Husmann.*)

A pain, as if a stitch would appear deep in the left side of the chest, posteriorly to the heart. (After two hours. *Geist.*)

Pain from the left side of the chest to the groins, increased by deep respiration, particularly in the groin and back; like a stitch. From 9 to 10 o'clock in the forenoon. (*Gosewisch.*)

RESPIRATION. Oppression in the chest on reclining, at the same time a trembling in the lower extremities. (B.)

315. Oppression in the upper part of the chest; not relieved by deep inspiration. (The 7th and following days. 3*d*. *Hering.*)

Difficulty of breathing; there seems to be an impediment in the region of the pit of the throat, and uppe part of the chest; at the same time itching pimples on the back and pain in the chest, below the point of the shoulder blade. (The 9th day. 3*d*. *Hering*.)

He often breathes deeply, as if the breast within and below was full, in the forenoon during sitting and writing. (The 11th day. 3*d*. *Hering*.)

The difficulty in his respiration in the depth of the chest, often returns in the afternoon and evening. (The 2d and 3d week. 3*d*. *Hering*.) Comp. 235.

Wheezing during respiration, observed more by others than himself, in the afternoon and evening; in the afternoon on the bed, on which occasion he has to turn backwards, if he wants to take a full breath. (The 6th week. 3*d*. *Hering*.)

320. * In two cases of incurable hydrothorax, fl. ac. gave much relief. (3*d*. *Jeanes*.)

HEART.—Uneasiness about the heart. (Immediately. 2*d*. *Neidhard*.)

Aching in region of heart. (After 15 minutes. 2*d*. *Neidhard*.)

Jerking in the heart. (After 1 hour. 2*d*. *Neidhard*.)

Painful jerking in the heart. (After 2 hours. 2*d*. *Neidhard*.)

325. Continual soreness in the heart. (After 1 hour. 2*d*. *Neidhard*.)

EXTERIOR CHEST.—Itching on the left breast and right side of the nose. After smelling. 30*th*. (*Husmann*.)

The severe itching on the breast, with small soft pimples, habitual to him in summer, is much increased on the 4th day. (3*d*. *Hering*.)

Slight pain close to the right nipple. (After 1 hour. 30*th*. *Gosewisch*.)

In the evening, itching on the right nipple and around it; the nipple is the next morning much larger, more red, and the areola darker. A thin brownish crust is formed on the areola. (The 12th and 13th day. 3*d*. *Hering*.)

NECK.—330. In the evening, during his walk, a very severe itching on the throat and chest. (The 10th day. 3*d*. *Hering*.)

In the forenoon pain in the right side of the neck. (6*th Freitag*.)

In the afternoon, violent drawing pain in the right side of the neck. (*Freitag*.)

Contraction in some muscles of the neck, on the left side and towards the shoulder, during the forenoon, on reposing and whilst rising. After some exercise it gradually subsides. The pain seems to change from one set of muscles to the other, but is always in more than one. The omohyoideus muscle is decidedly affected. (4th day. 3*d*. *Hering*.)

Rigidity in the nape of the neck, soon after taking it. (5 o'clock, P. M. 5*th*. *Williamson*.)

335. Sorēness in the left half of the nape. (1st day. 5*th*. *Williamson*.)

Very transient drawing pain along the right side of the nape. (5*th*. *Williamson*.)

Now and then warm flushes like a warm breath, from the nape of the neck towards the occiput. (Lasting 8 days. 30*th*. *Husmann*.)

Warm streamings from the right nape to the shoulder. Comp. 496.

Headache, from the nape of the neck through the centre of the head, towards the forehead, dull pressure. Comp. 50.

BACK.—Strong heat, extending from the centre of the dorsal region to the loins. (After 3 hours. *Campos*.)

Deep seated pain in the left lumbar region at night. (4th day. 2*d*. *Williamson*.)

340. A pain under the point of the right shoulder blade, to which he was formerly subject, and which impels him to bend the body backwards and to stretch; appears after a few hours, and returns occasionally for several days; but more rarely after some weeks. (3*d*. *Hering*.)

Deep seated pain in the back, below the point of the shoulder-blade, more towards the left; it occurs more in a sitting posture, particularly whilst riding. (The 4th and 9th day. 3*d*. *Hering*.)

Pain in the back, sometimes high up near the shoulder-blades, sometimes deeply seated, as it were in the region of the kidneys. (1st week. 3*d*. *Hering*.)

Violent itching, and small pimples on both shoulders and on the back, more towards the left. (11th and following days. 3*d*. *Hering*.)

* His habitual bruised pain in os sacrum and lumbar region, (relieved by stretching and bending backwards, but particularly by pressure, as well after fatiguing bodily labour,) is much aggravated by fl. ac. 6*th*, but is removed entirely after fl. ac. 30*th;* a similar pain, however, returns in the region of the right shoulder, which is also quickly cured after a dose of fl. ac. 3*d*, it returns during the 4th and 5th day, in the back below, between and above the shoulder, and only disappears in the 2d week. (*Hering*.)

345. Aching pain in the os sacrum, very soon. (2*d*. *Neidhard*.)

Jerkings in sacrum, during the 1st hour, and less frequently the 2d hour. (2*d*. *Neidhard*.)

Pricking, burning, itching near the os coccygis, towards the right. (4th day. 3*d*. *Hering*.)

UPPER EXTREMITIES.—Creeping and severe itching on the right shoulder. (Evening, after 5 or 6 hours. 3*d*. *Hering*.)

In the evening, changing from the top of one shoulder to the other; severe itching, with now and then a single stitch in the skin. (1st day. 3*d*. *Hering*.)

350. In the afternoon violent itching on the left shoulder, in the evening on the back, where small pimples arise; worse late at night until he falls asleep. (The 4th and 5th day. 3*d*. *Hering*.)

Burning pricking pain in the left shoulder-blade. (After 1 or 2 hours. 3*d*. *Hering*.)

Sudden jerking pain in the left shoulder, in the bone. (*Freitag.*)

Pain in the left shoulder, beneath the skin; and in the left side of the chest. Comp. 304.

Pain of a deeply penetrating character, first in the right, afterwards in the left arm, most about the junction of the cancellated with the solid portion of the os humeri; even after the disappearance of the pain, there is soreness upon pressure of the parts previously affected. A similar pain in the muscles over the head of the left radius. (In 40 minutes. 3*d.* *Jeanes.*)

Rheumatic pain in the bones of the left arm, from elbow to shoulder, with lameness. (After 1 hour. 2*d.* *Neidhard.*)

355. In the afternoon pain in the right upper arm in the bone towards the elbow. From the right arm the pain passed over to the left arm, with the same pain in bone. (2d day. 2*d.* *Neidhard.*)

In the forenoon at 9 o'clock pressing pain in the right arm, and a constriction in the left side of the neck. (*Freitag.*)

In the morning a pressing pain in the left arm, just above the elbow. (6*th.* *Freitag.*)

Pain in the left arm above the elbow, appearing after the pains on the right side. (After 1 or 2 hours. 3*d.* *Hering.*)

Trembling in the biceps of the right arm. (After 15 minutes. 2*d.* *Williamson.*)

360. Trembling in the triceps of the right arm. (5th day. 2*d.* *Williamson.*)

Aching in the right elbow joint. (2d day. 2*d.* *Williamson.*)

Aching in the left elbow, in the evening. (4th day. 2*d.* *Williamson.*)

During the pain in the left side a pain in the right elbow-joint. (*Geist.*)

In the middle of the left forearm a slight pinching pain; lasting only a short time. (In the evening. 1*st.* *E. Smith.*)

365. Aching pains in the bones of the left forearm, towards the middle. (2*d.* *Neidhard.*)

A pain in the right shoulder-joint, which he had felt a week before last, but not the last; returned for a few moments, and *extended towards the fingers, as if air was passing down*, a sensation which he had never experienced before. (After 1 hour. *Geist.*)

A burning, pricking and jerking pain in the whole left arm, often returning, as if there was passing through the nerves a very painful, but slow electric shock. Most severe he feels it on the inside of the left little finger, together with now and then a sharp stitch in the point of the finger, passing fiom within outwardly. (In the afternoon, 2 o'clock, 2d day. 30*th.* *Hering.*)

An almost painful electric jerk, along the left radius to the thumb, which moves involuntarily. (Several times at 12 o'clock, 2d day. 3*d.* *Hering.*)

In the evening at 10 o'clock, the right arm, on which he rests, becomes benumbed and feels lame, with a pricking sensation. (3*d.* *Hering.*)

Slight lameness in the right arm, so thathe has some difficulty in writing. (After 15 minutes. 2*d.* *Neidhard.*)

370. Pressure and lameness, with pain in the forearm. 453.

Heaviness in the right arm, in the morning on awaking, with some numbness, although he only laid on the left side. (2d day. 30*th.* *Husmann.*)

On awaking, the right upper arm and shoulder feel bruised and benumbed, after lying on left side. (After several days. 30*th.* *Hering.*)

The left forearm and hand as if asleep, at 5 o'clock, A. M., whilst lying on the right side. (7th day. 2*d.* *Williamson.*)

The left hand is asleep in the morning, and remains so the whole forenoon. (2d day. 3*d.* *Hering.*)

375. A sensation of numbness in the left hand, extending to the forearm; the sensation is different from the numbness produced by long pressure, and also more

lasting, and does not subside after using exertion. (2d day. 3*d*. *Hering*.)

Sensation of numbness, jerking and lameness in the left arm, appears in the morning and forenoon, and subsides again between 12 and 1 o'clock. (3*d*. *Hering*.)

The numbness and paralytic sensation in the left forearm, returns every forenoon, but every day at a later period, and less decided. (4th, also the 10th and 11th day. 3*d*. *Hering*.) Comp. 318.

Numb pain in the forearms to the hand. (6*th*. *Freitag*.)

Lameness of the right hand. (30*th*. *Freitag*.)

380. Powerless sensation in the hands. (B.)

Weakness and numbness in the head and hands. 83.

In the fingers of the right hand some numbness and rigidity. (In the forenoon. 30*th*. *Husmann*.)

Drawing in the right wrist in the forearm from 8 to 11 o'clock. (6th day. *Pehrson*.)

Pain about the right wrist and finger-joints. (After 1 hour. 3*d*. *Jeanes*.)

After a cold from exposure, pain in the right metacarpus. (In the evening. 6*th*. *Hering*.)

385. Both hands are constantly very red. (3d and following days. 3*d*. *Hering*.)

The hands are full and warm, uncommonly red, particularly in the palms, and like marbled. (4th day. 3*d*. *Hering*.)

Heat in the palm of the right hand. (The succeeding forenoon. 30*th*. *Husmann*.)

* A perspiration in the palms of the hands, (even during cold dry weather, and with the back of the hand dry and cool; his palms were constantly so moist that every one who shook hands with him observed it,) which remained after lobelia; disappeared the 4th day of the fl. ac. proving. (*Geist*.)

On the right index finger violent itching and small vesicles. (Evening, the 5th day. 3*d*. *Hering*.)

390. Pain in the first joint of the right little finger,

as if it were being pulled out of joint. (After 15 minutes. *2d. Williamson.*)

Burning around the first bone of the right middle finger, together with an itching, stinging in the skin. (After 1 hour. *3d. Hering.*)

Pain in the left index finger, as it were in the bone, now and then during the day, the whole finger is painful interiorly, particularly in the evening. (5th day. *3d. Hering.*)

Aching in the left index finger. (6th day. *2d. Williamson.*)

Acute prickings, like with a needle, in the fingers. (*6th. Freitag.*)

395. Pricking in the ends of the index fingers, most in the left; also in the right thumb. (4th day. *2d. Williamson.*)

Jerking in the left thumb occasionally, extending to the middle of the forearm. (During the forenoon. *3d. Hering.*)

Now and then a pain resembling a contusion in the ends of several fingers, as it were in the bones. (In the evening the 4th and following weeks. *3d. Hering.*)

A violent burning stitch in the fleshy part of the left thumb; often returning and passing out at the end. (11 o'clock, A. M., 2d day. *3d. Hering.*)

Painless sensation beneath the nail of the left thumb, as if something was working gradually its way out. (2d day, A. M. *3d. Hering.*)

400. Slowly jerking, repeated burning in the end of the left little finger. (10 o'clock, A. M. 2d day. *3d. Hering.*)

During the forenoon, until 2 o'clock, sensation of a pain along the back of the left little finger, he repeatedly looks, if it is not actually there. (7th week. *3d. Hering.*)

During the 6th week there yet arise larger and smaller vesicles, in groups, with very sensitive itching on the ulnar side of the right thumb, and the radial side of the index finger, leaving behind them dry scurfy spots. (3*d.* *Hering.*)

Soreness of warts on the left hand. (2*d.* *Esrey.*)

For several weeks the growth of the nails seems to be much more rapid. (3*d.* *Hering.*)

LOWER EXTREMITIES.—405. Acute stitches on the right hip bone, spreading themselves over the glutëi muscles. (After 1 hour. *Geist.*)

Pain in the right hip. (After 45 minutes. 3*d.* *Jeanes.*)

Pain in the inner condyle of the left femur. (80 minutes. 3*d.* *Jeanes.*)

Lameness in the left hip. (2d day. 2*d.* *Williamson.*)

Soreness and pain, on motion, in the left hip, particularly felt on getting in or out of bed; worse in the morning. (3d day. 2*d.* *Williamson.*)

410. Pain in the right ischiatic nerve. (Afternoon. 30*th.* *Husmann.*)

A violent, slightly burning, quick, nervous pain proceeds from the region of the bladder, down to the right thigh, whilst lying in bed. (1st day. 6*th.* *Hering.*)

Burning, shooting pain, as if it were in the nerve, from the right hip downwards, particularly on the inside of the knee; farther down less distinctly. (2d day. *Hering.*)

Pressing pain in the fleshy part of left thigh on the outside. (*Geist.*)

Burning, itching pain in the back part of the thigh. (After smelling. 30*th.* *Husmann.*)

415. Soreness in the muscles of the thighs. (2d day. 2*d.* *Williamson.*)

Bruise-like pain of the thigh, particularly in the posterior and inner portion. (2d and 3d day. 3*d.* *Hering.*)

Pain on the inside of the right knee, in the evening. (After 15 minutes. 2*d.* *Williamson.*)

Penetrating pain on the outside of the left knee. (4th day. 2*d.* *Williamson.*)

Dead feeling in the right knee-joint. (1st day. *E. Smith.*)

420. Pain in the right knee-joint; also pain in bones of right forearm. (After 4 hours. 2*d*. *Neidhard.*)

Deep-seated pain below the right knee. (In the evening, after 15 minutes. 2*d*. *Williamson.*)

Severe pain in the left knee, on the outside, disappears after friction. (Evening, 8 o'clock. *Geist.*)

Drawing pain in the calf of the right leg, beginning at the hollow of the knee, and extending to the tendon achilles. (The next forenoon. 30*th*. *Husmann.*)

Drawing pain in the left leg and foot. (*Freitag.*)

425. Tearing pain in the right knee from below upwards; after that a quick, very transient pressing pain in the left temple. (30*th*. *Husmann.*)

Right foot quite lame, and a dull aching pain in the os femoris, tibia and fibula. (2*d*. *Neidhard.*)

In the evening slight numbness of the right thigh, only whilst crossing the legs. (In 3 hours. 3*d*. *Hering.*)

The left leg falls easily asleep. (The 9th and 10th day. 3*d*. *Hering.*)

In the evening during a walk, drawing pain in the right ankle-joint, spreads gradually over the whole leg, producing a lameness in the knee and ankle, so that he is hardly able to proceed; it disappears during rest, but returns on renewing his walk, when it also affects the right ankle-joint. (6th day. The same pain and weakness during walking, also on the 7th day, but in a less degree. *Pehrson.*)

430. In the afternoon, for a quarter of an hour, a sensation of lameness, like a sprain, in the right ankle-joint; it passes all around the joint, and is very painful at each step, after walking and resting for a while it gradually disappears. (After having taken a small dose of tinct. colchicum.) (30*th*. *Hering.*)

Sprain-like pain in the left ankle-joint during walking. (16th day. 3*d*. *Hering.*)

Pressing pain in the left foot. (*Freitag.*)

Pain in the right external ankle. (Evening after 15 minutes. *Williamson.*)

Pain and burning in the right instep. (3 hours. 3*d.* *Jeanes.*)

435. A pain in the left instep. (Evening, in 2 hours. 3*d.* *Hering.*)

Itching in the left instep. (From smelling. 30*th.* *Husmann.*)

Heat in the sole of the right foot. (After 15 minutes. 2*d.* *Williamson.*)

Crawling sensation in the sole of the right foot. (4th day. 2*d.* *Williamson.*)

Burning feeling in the sole of the right foot. (In 2 hours. *Jeanes.*)

440. In the morning, burning stitches under the soles of both feet. (The 15th day. *Pehrson.*)

Violent burning pain in all the toes, so that he could hardly walk. (After 3 and 4 hours. 2*d.* *Neidhard.*)

Severe pains in all the left toes except the large, after the 8th dose. (6*th.* *Freitag.*)

Pain in the toes of the right foot in the first joints. (After three hours. 3*d.* *Jeanes.*)

Very acute pricking pain in the ends of the toes of the right foot. (The next forenoon. 30*th.* *Husmann.*)

445. (On the second toe of the left foot a painful excoriation, which apparently bleeds.) (After 3 hours. 2*d.* *Neidhard.*)

Pain in the corns of the right foot. (2*d.* *Esrey.*)

Soreness of all his corns, like a bile. (After 3 hours. 2*d.* *Neidhard.*)

GENERAL SYMPTOMS.—Sensation, as if the shoulder and hip-joints were going to be pulled out of joint. *Campos.*)

Jerking pains in different parts of the body, behind the left ear, on the left middle finger and in os sacrum. (During the 1st hour. 2*d.* *Neidhard.*)

450. Violent jerking, burning pains, confined to a small space. (3*d.* *Hering.*)

Slight erratic pain in the left half of the body, in the

arm, chest, thigh, etc., with a sensation of slight itching. (After half an hour. *Geist.*)

Pains of a short duration, in the left leg, arm, and hand. (After the 8th dose. *6th. Freitag.*)

Pressure and sensation of lameness, particularly in the hand, arm to the elbow, and in the foot. (*6th. Freitag.*)

In the evening pressing pain in different parts of short duration; on the chin, neck, in the right forearm, in the left knee, right foot, also in the right shoulder; and left arm at times below, at others above the elbow. (*Freitag.*)

455. Different aching pains in the bones of the forearms and legs about the centre, going and coming. (*2d. Neidhard.*)

While sitting, pleasurable movements of the whole body, unawares. (*Campos.*)

Hands, fingers, toes, feet, jaws, lips, eyebrows and lids, muscles of the face, etc., all are in motion. (In 10 hours. *Campos.*)

Increased ability to exercise his muscles without fatigue, regardless of the most excessive heat* in summer, or cold in winter; he is able to perform with the greatest facility, his usual daily walk of several miles, which every day previously he thought very fatiguing and annoying. (*Campos.*)

Walking is difficult, because the legs feel tired; he is hardly able to drag them along; they are so heavy that he finds it necessary to hold on to the arm of some one else for support. (*Campos.*)

460. In the evening, very suddenly, an unusual very great tiredness. (*Geist.*)

Excessively languid. (In the forenoon after second dose. *2d. Williamson.*)

Is less tired than usual after a walk in the evening. (The 8th and 11th day. *3d. Hering.*)

SLEEP.—He is unusually wakeful in the evening. (8th day. *3d. Hering.*)

* The prover resides in Norfolk, Va., situated 36° 50′ of latitude.

Sleeplessness, scarcely any inclination to sleep. (*Campos.*)

465. *No desire to sleep.* (*Campos.*)

Day or night without his usual sleep, he feels as if he had already slept. (*Campos.*)

Sleeplessness from the time he has gone to bed until near morning, when a very short and light sleep will be sufficient to refresh him, as if he had slept all night. (*Campos.*)

Drowsiness, constant sleepiness, for the first five days after the acid. (*Campos.*)

In the morning, soon after taking the acid, unconquerable sleepiness; after a short and refreshing sleep, it nevertheless returns every two hours until evening. (*Pehrson.*)

470. Every forenoon about 10 to 12 o'clock he becomes sleepy and tired. (During the 1st week. 3*d*. *Hering.*)

Periodical attacks of sleepiness in the afternoon of the second day. (*Pehrson.*)

In the evening, earlier, sleepy. (During the first two weeks. 3*d*. *Hering.*)

Sudden sleepiness in the evening. (The 5th, 7th, 8th, 10th, and 12th day. 3*d*. *Hering.*)

Profound sleep until late in the morning. (During 1st week, for several days. 3*d*. *Hering.*)

475. Soon after falling asleep, anxious, frightful dreams, with waking up at midnight; the rest of the night, many dreams of distant acquaintances, in a person who almost never dreams. (1st day. *Pehrson.*)

Dreams of distant acquaintances and things. (The whole of the 2d night. *Pehrson.*)

Many dreams for 15 nights, quite unusual. (*Pehrson.*)

All his dreams were very lucid, as if they really happened, and although they were sometimes disagreeable, they were never vexatious. (*Pehrson.*)

He dreams of the sudden death of his friends, and

severely reproaches himself for neglecting them. (1st day. 6*th*. *Hering*.)

480. Dreams that he was dead, and orders the rapid removal of the corpse out of the house. (B.)

A very vivid dream; sees his nearest relatives die. (2d day. 30*th*. *Husmann*.)

Restless nights, dreams easy to remember, of the occurrences of the day, in a person who has not dreamed for years. (12*th*. *Gosewisch*.)

The whole night very vivid dreams, with minuteness of detail. He forgets them soon after awaking. (After several days. 20*th*. *Hering*.)

Restless nights, with many dreams, which he cannot recollect. (2*d*. *Neidhard*.)

485. Dreams, particularly towards morning, and generally of a frightful character. (*Freitag*.)

Many dreams, but only after midnight. (7th day. *Pehrson*.)

Dreams towards morning. (For the first time on the 9th and 10th day. 3*d*. *Hering*.)

Snoring in his sleep and exclamations in the dream. (6*th*. *Hering*.)

Thirst in the night. (*Campos*.)

490. Notwithstanding going to bed very late, he awakes frequently, and has many dreams; yet he wakes very early in the morning and feels better than usual. (During the 1st week. 3*d* and 6*th*. *Hering*.)

HEAT.—Sensation as if a burning vapour was emitted from the pores of the whole body. (*Campos*.)

The first evening, and still more during the next morning, a sensation of greater warmth in the body; cold bathing is more than ordinarily agreeable. (The 1st and the following day, but less. 3*d*. *Hering*.)

* He can bear the summer heat much better, and feels less lassitude than usual. (For several weeks. 3*d*. *Hering*.

General heat after little exercise. (The 1st evening. 3*d*. *Hering*.)

495. General feeling of heat, heaviness and lameness of the whole body. (After 1 hour. *2d.* *Neidhard.*)

PERSPIRATION.—Perspiration and sensation of heat on the upper part of the body towards the right, particularly along the right of the nape of neck towards the shoulder, like in warm streams. (Evening from 7 to 8 o'clock. 2d day. 30*th.* *Husmann.*)

Profuse, sour, offensive *perspiration.* (Afternoon. *2d.* *Williamson.*)

For several evenings an unusually profuse and glutinous perspiration, with itching. (3*d.* *Hering.*) Compare 1.

SKIN.—Burning pains on small spots of the skin, on the back part of the right hand, angle of the index finger, and here and there on the left hand. (30*th.* *Hering.*)

500. Burning more externally, in different places, but always on one spot; on the right thigh; left upper arm, left thigh, etc. Also on the fingers. (Evening, 9 o'clock, after the 4th dose. *Geist.*)

A slight glow on the lower part of the right buttock, towards the anterior. (Evening. 30*th.* *Hering.*)

Itching on the left shin, on the left glutei muscles and forehead. (*Geist.*)

A group of small red pimples, on the left hip, in the back part of the joint, and below on a spot half as large as the palm of the hand; which have opened during the night after scratching. (4th and following days. 3*d.* *Hering.*)

Itching all over in different places, but for the most part in the posterior parts. (For 5 weeks. 3*d.* *Hering.*)

505. The itching is most severe and lasts longest on back. (3*d.* *Hering.*)

The itching is always worse in the evening. (3*d.* *Hering.*)

Itching the whole day, in different spots, particularly on the back. (4th day. 3*d.* *Hering.*)

Violent pricking, itching on detached spots, mostly on the left side, particularly on the side of the chest towards the back, and on the thigh in the evening, about

10 to 11 o'clock. (Third and following days. 3*d*. *Hering*.)

Itching on the left side of the nape of the neck, on top and below the shoulder, and on the back, every evening and morning. (The 4th and following days. 3*d*. *Hering*.)

510. Violent itching, and small pimples here and there. (6*th*. *Hering*.)

* The itching of the skin habitual to him in the month of March, disappears. (6*th*. *Hering*.)

Violent itching on the cicatrice of an old abscess, on the inside of the left thigh. (Third day. 3*d*. *Hering*.)

Itching of all cicatrices in the evening; they are all on the left side; on the thigh, upper arm, and the most recent on the left hand, cut by glass; this last itches most severely. (Third day. 3*d*. *Hering*.)

The 4th morning *all his cicatrices*, dating from thirty-two to two years, *are red around the edges*, and occupied here and there with itching vesicles. Those of more ancient date, have larger vesicles; those of late date are filled with very small pimples, but only on the tissue of the cicatrice, and not on the surrounding skin. 3*d*. *Hering*.)

515. Elevated red blotches (above the eyebrows, most abundant on the left side, but of longer continuation on the right) still continue, whilst the other symptoms disappear. (Evening of 4th day. *Williamson*.)

Pimples on the abdomen, but principally on the thighs and legs, the points of which formed a crust the next day, after taking fl. ac., and which scaled off the 17th day after taking the first dose, and the 8th day after the 4th dose. (*Freitag*.)

Several small light carmine red, round, elevated, blood vesicles, resembling little flesh-warts; they are very soft and compressible, and by a strong and steady pressure the blood disappears, but immediately returns again. The largest is the size of a hempseed, the smaller ones like millet seeds; some are still smaller, but they are very perceptible as light red enlargements of the capillaries, raising up the cuticle. The largest is an inch below the right nipple; and the same distance towards the right of it, a smaller one, one inch below the same nipple; two on the right side of the median line of the abdomen above the navel; a still smaller one on the right side of the chest; five very small ones of light colour, on the inside of the right upper and lower arm.

He noticed them for the first time about the 13th day. Three weeks later some of the smaller ones had disappeared. The larger had become darker, somewhat resembling nævi materni; those above the navel are also larger. After three months they are paler. They made their appearance and remained without any itching. (3*d*. *Hering*.)

* Numerous varicose veins of 20 years standing on the left leg of an old man, are diminished one half, after repeated doses of fluoric acid. (12*th*. *Neidhard*.)

ACIDUM OXALICUM.

BY C. NEIDHARD, M. D.

OXALIC Acid; *Kleesaeure;* Germ.—discovered by Scheele, in the year 1783, by the decomposition of sugar with strong nitric acid, which he first considered as saccharine acid, but afterwards found it identical with oxalic acid.

Preparation. The excess of acid in the binoxalate of potassa is neutralized by the carbonate of potassa, and the neutral oxalate is decomposed by the acetate of lead. In consequence of a double decomposition, a precipitate of oxalate of lead is obtained. This is to be well washed and dried, and decomposed by means of one-third of its weight of strong sulphuric acid, previously diluted with ten times of its weight of water. An insoluble sulphate of lead is formed, and the oxalic acid being liberated, may be made to crystallize by evaporation. The mother waters, by fresh evaporation, furnish fresh portions of crystals, until quite exhausted. By this process a very pure acid may be obtained.*

* Drs. Wood and Bache American Dispensatory. Appendix.

Its purity may readily be tested by dissolving it in a sufficient quantity of water, adding carbonate of lime cautiously, until effervescence ceases, filtering, drying the precipitated oxalate of lime, and observing that, for every hundred grains of oxalic acid, if pure, there should be a product of about two hundred and five grains of oxalate. As, however, in operating on a small quantity, a slight difference of weight, which might be produced by the presence of tartrate of lime along with the oxalate in the precipitate, might not be observed, the purity of the acid may be still more satisfactorily ascertained by digesting the supposed oxalate of lime in a solution of tartaric acid, and again drying it. Should any tartrate have been present, it will have been taken up by the acid solution, which will be indicated by the loss of weight in the precipitate.—*American Journal of Pharmacy.*

Many substances yield oxalic acid, by the action of nitric acid; *e. g.*, it is obtained by the decomposition of honey, manna and other sweet juices of herbs, most of the essential and fixed oils, and even the animal gelatin. Fifteen parts of the oil of sassafras furnish one-part of pure crystallized oxalic acid.

According to L. Gmelin and Liebig it is also formed during the preparation of potash; and according to Vauquelin and Gay-Lussac, if gelatinous or pectic acid is heated in a crucible with caustic potash or soda, and the mass is dissolved in dilute nitric acid. In the same manner oxalic acid may be obtained from cotton, silk, hair, tendons, wool, also from the coagulum of blood and white of eggs, wood shavings, sugar, starch, gum, sugar of milk, paper, and other organic substances; vegetable substances by decomposition with potash. M. Berthollet remarks, that the quantity of oxalic acid furnished by vegetable matters, is proportionate to their nutritive quality, and particularly of that from cotton, he could not obtain any sensible quantity. Whether this is correct, remains to be seen. One of the most remarkable formations of it remains, that of tartaric acid; even the crude tartar furnishes, heated with potash, a great quantity of oxalic acid. Citric, malic acid, the acid of amber, cherries, currants, raspberries, furnish it. Those organic matters, as sugar and starch, which contain oxygen and hydrogen in the same proportion as water, yield it in the greatest quantity. It is generated occasionally in consequence of diseased action in the kidneys, and deposited in the bladder as an oxalate of lime, forming a peculiar concretion, called from its appearance the mulberry calculus. It is also found in the liquor allantoidis of the cow.

In natuie, oxalic acid is never found in the pulp of fruits, but often in combination with potash in the cellular tissue, (Zellstoffe) of the leaves, *e. g.* of Oxalis acetosella corniculata, cornua, L. (woodsorrell); stricta Jacq.; floribunda, L.; tetraphylla, E., of Mexico, the leaves of which are a remedy for the scurvy.* Again, Rumex acetosa, L., (common sorrell,) Rumex vesicar., Geranium acetosum, etc., contain oxalic acid ; a similar taste have the leaves of the begonia, of the tree acetosa, Rumph. and several exotic plants. Particularly rich of *oxalate of lime* is the Asiatic lichen Parmelia esculenta; also the cellular tissue of the marrow and the bark of Cereus peruvianus. This oxydized acid (oxydirte saeure) always seems to be most predominant in that part of the plant which is most exposed to the air, and which seems appropriate for the attraction of the oxygen from it. Oxalate of lime lies as a powder in the perennial roots and barks of many annual plants, *e. g.* the rhubarb, red gentian, liquorice, clove, and other roots. According to Braconnot, the Lichenes crustacei, like variolaria, (to be found on old beech trees) are almost half composed of oxalate of lime, whilst in the more frequent tuberculous lichens it does not occur at all.† Oxalic acid, in combination with the protoxide of iron, constitutes the mineral denominated by Rivero Humboldtine, by Necker and Beudant Humboldtite. In a *free state* it is said to be secreted from the tubelike, but not from the glandular hairs on the delicate husks and chalices of the Cicer aristenum, (chickpea.) Pereira, however, is doubtful of the accuracy of the statement.

A principal means of detecting oxalic acid and the oxalates, is afforded by their deportment with concentrated sulphuric acid ; crystallized oxalic acid, as well as its salts, dissolve in concentrated sulphuric acid at an elevated temperature, and this solution, upon continued application of heat, evolves, with all the phenomena usually attendant upon boiling a gas, which burns with a blue flame, and produces in lime water a precipitate

* Gay-Lussac in Schweigger—Seidel's Jahrb. 1830, 1 heft; in Geiger's Magazin fuer Pharmacie, etc:, 1831, xxxv. page 28; and in Annalen der Pharmacie, 1832, i. 1, page 20; also Buchner and Herberger's Repertorium, 1831, xxxvii., 2, p. 189.

† Annal. de Chimie, Mars 1825, and Trommsdorff eues Journ. der Pharm. 1825, xi., 1.

of lime; this gas consists of a mixture of equal volumes of carbonic oxide gas and carbonic acid gas. No charring of the oxalic acid nor evolution of sulphurous acid, occurs in this decomposition. Other organic acids, such as citric acid, formic acid, etc. etc., evolve likewise carbonic oxide gas upon being heated with sulphuric acid; but citric acid gets charred in the operation, and the process moreover is attended with evolution of sulphurous acid; whilst the carbonic oxide gas evolved from formic acid—which undergoes no charring in the operation—is pure from any admixture of carbonic acid gas. This method (heating with concentrated sulphuric acid) affords us, therefore, a simple and certain means of detecting oxalic acid and distinguishing it from all other organic acids.*

Oxalic acid is a white crystallized salt, in the shape of slender, flattened, four or six-sided prisms, with two sided summits. When exposed to a very dry atmosphere, it undergoes a slight efflorescence. Its crystals are more or less transparent and tolerably bright, without odour, of an exceedingly acrid but not disagreeably sour taste. Of all organic acids, oxalic acid has the greatest amount of acidity; one part imparts to 200,000 parts of water an acid taste. Its specific weight is, according to Guyton-Morveau 1.593, according to Richter 1.507. It dissolves in about nine times its weight of cold, and its own weight of boiling water. The solution takes place with a slight crepitation. It dissolves also, but not to the same extent, in alcohol. One hundred parts of boiling alcohol dissolve fifty-six parts of oxalic acid; in a medium temperature, only forty parts. It forms with alcohol the oxalic ether. The acid dissolved in alcohol reddens litmus more readily than the other acids, and Fernambucco paper is rendered pale-yellow more rapidly; turmeric paper, however, remains unchanged.

Composition.—Oxalic acid consists of two equiva-

* Liebig's Lectures on Organic Chemistry in London Lancet.

lents of carbon, 12.24, and three oxygen, 24 = 36.24. Two equivalents of this water may be driven off by a regulated heat, by which the acid is made to effloresce, but the third cannot be expelled without destroying the acid itself. Accordingly, as in the case of nitric acid, we have no knowledge of anhydrous oxalic acid in an uncombined state.

From the constitution of oxalic acid, as above given, it is plain that this acid corresponds in composition to carbonic acid and oxide taken together, and is, therefore, intermediate in the quantity of oxygen, which it contains, between this acid and oxide. Notwithstanding it contains less oxygen than carbonic acid, it is incomparably stronger as an acid, which circumstance may be accounted for by supposing some peculiarity in the mode in which its constituents are combined.*

Brugnatelli speaks highly favourable of oxalic acid as a test for uric acid in stones of the bladder. According to Doebereiner, it forms a quickly acting test for the oxides of cobalt and nickel, as these are powerfully attracted by it.

Chemical affinities.—Oxalic acid has the greatest affinity for lime, and lime reciprocally for oxalic acid. This is the case also in double elective affinities, so that sulphate, nitrate, muriate and acetate of lime are decomposed by the oxalate of lime; and as soon as it is combined with these salts, oxalate of lime is precipitated. On this account oxalic acid or binoxalate of potash is a very useful reagent on lime in any water. The degree of their affinity is in the following order: barytes, strontian, magnesia, potash, and soda, glycine, alumina, forming simple oxalic salts.

In all these salts the acid is decomposed by a heat exceeding the boiling point of water, so that only carbonate of potash, soda, etc., is left. In the case of the oxalate of ammonium, the latter becomes partly volatilized as ammonium, partly in the state of carbonate of ammonia.

* Wood and Bache, American Dispensatory. Appendix.

In the degree of its affinity to the alkalies, oxalic acid comes immediately after sulphüric acid; for lime and magnesia it has, however, a greater affinity than the latter. This forms the distinction between oxalic and tartaric acid, as the latter comes after sulphuric acid in its affinity for lime. With regard to barytes and alumine, sulphuric acid takes the precedence of oxalic acid. Oxalic acid has also less affinity for the alkalies than nitric and hydrochloric acid, but more than they, for lime, barytes and magnesia; of fluoric and boracic acid it generally takes the precedence. Phosphoric acid, on the other hand, has a greater affinity for the alkalies, but a lesser for the earths than oxalic acid, as is also the case with tartaric acid.

Oxalic acid has the same tendency to unite itself with the vegetable alkali in the same proportion as the tartaric acid with the tartrate of potash.

It will not be deemed inappropriate to give in this place an account of oxalium, the *quadroxalate of potash*, synon. bioxalas kalicus, kali oxalicum acidulum, sal acetosellae, commonly called salt of sorrel.

It is obtained by crystallizing one part of oxalic acid, with carbonate of potash, and adding to the solution three parts more of acid. It crystallizes in colourless transparent prisms of the doubly oblique prismatic system; and which consist of 4 equiv. oxalic acid 144.129. Potash 48 and 7 equiv. water 36=255. If three parts of the salt be converted into carbonate by heat, and added to a solution of one part, the neutral oxalate of potash is formed. (*Liebig.*)

The commercial quadroxalate is not pure, for Pereira found that it yields, by ignition in a covered crucible, carbonate of potash, contaminated with carbonaceous matter; whereas the pure quadroxalate yields the carbonate only. It is employed for removing ink stains and iron moulds from linen, and for decolourizing straw, used for bonnet making. This salt was formerly used in medicine, as a refrigerant. In France, tablettes ou pastilles la soif, are prepared with it. It possesses poisonous properties similar to, but less energetic than oxalic acid.*

Experiments on Animals.

The most extensive experiments with oxalic acid were performed by Drs. Christison and Coindet, read in a memoir on the subject, before the Medico-Chirurgical Society of Edinburgh, Feb. 5, 1823. They chose them from a list of nearly forty cases, and they are described very nearly in the same words as those employed in the original reports, taken while the animal was under the action of the poison. Unfortunately they are only of a conditional value as elucidating the pure physiological effect of oxalic acid, as in some instances the acid was introduced into the stomach, by an aperture made into the œsophagus, and retained by a ligature. In others, half an inch of the pneumogastric and sympathetic nerves was removed. It was also injected into the pleura; the peritoneum, and the intestines were tied in several places. They themselves acknowledge that some of the effects ought to be ascribed to those somewhat forcible proceedings. For the homœopathic observer, they are, however, particularly interesting, as tending to show, that this poison acts neither by its corrosive effect on the stomach, and secondarily on the nerves and brain, nor by its absorption into the blood alone, but, as will be elucidated by our experiments on the healthy, in its own way, uninfluenced by any theories for the purpose of establishing certain premises.

In the following pages we have endeavoured to embody into our article the most essential points of their labours, giving in the majority of instances a detailed account of the experiments, as they are to be found in the original treatise.

Dr. Christison and Coindet engaged in them for the ostensible purpose of ascertaining the correctness of the views of Royston, Dr. Thompson and others, who main-

* Pereira Materia Medica, Vol. I, page 309.

tained that the acid and the membranes of the stomach mutually decompose one another; that a part of it enters the circulation, because the blood in various places reddens litmus; that these phenomena, however, are insufficient to account for death, and that its proximate cause is the injury done to *the heart and brain*, which are sympathetically affected by the injury done the stomach.

After their numerous experiments, they arrived at the following conclusions:

1. Oxalic acid, when introduced into the stomach in large doses, and highly concentrated, irritates it or corrodes it, by dissolving the gelatin of its coats, and death takes place by a sympathetic injury of the nervous system.

2. When diluted, it acts neither by irritating the stomach, nor by sympathy, but through the medium of absorption upon distant organs; and ceteris paribus, *it acts much more readily when diluted, than when concentrated.*

3. Though it is absorbed, it cannot be detected in any of the fluids, because probably it undergoes decomposition in passing through the lungs, and its elements combine with blood.

4. It is a direct sedative. (?) The organs it acts upon are the spine and the brain primarily, and the lungs and heart secondarily; and the immediate cause of death is sometimes paralysis of the heart, sometimes slow asphyxia, and sometimes a combination of both.

Experiment 1st.

For the purpose of ascertaining the *action of oxalic acid* as a *corrosive poison*, half an ounce of it in twice its weight of water, about 130° F., was injected into the stomach of a dog, by an aperture in the œsophages, and retained by a ligature. In two minutes he was seized with violent efforts to vomit, which continued till the 12th minute. The breathing was increased in fulness and frequency. In sixteen minutes and a half it became short, and occasionally suspended for a few seconds. At the same time he hung the head, looked very dull, but continued quite sensible. At last he fell suddenly on his side, the body was spasmodically extended for a few seconds, then completely relaxed, and after a few convulsive gasps, he died *twenty-one minutes* from the beginning of the experiment. During these convulsive gasps no pulse could be felt in the chest, and on opening the body immediately after the last of them, the heart was found not contractile, its right cavities much distended with dark blood, while that in the left was small in quantity and very florid.

The stomach was cut open and washed four minutes after death. Externally it was somewhat vascular. It contained a few ounces of a thick dark-brown oily-like matter. The internal surface was lined with mucus not inspissated. The epidermis of the villous coat was removed from the whole of the cardiac region, and from the posterior surface, and in patches only from the anterior; where it still remained, it was brittle, less adherent and of a brownish yellow colour. The posterior surface showed considerable vascularity, and streaks of black granular extravasation, confined to the corion of the villous coat. The internal membrane of the œsophagus below the ligature was corrugated, greyish coloured, but strong. All the other organs were healthy.

This experiment was often repeated by them in similar circumstances, and uniformly with analogous results, varying only in intensity. The violence of the efforts to vomit, has been directly proportioned to the quantity of the poison; when very violent, they cease sooner, when less frequent or violent, they sometimes lasted above two hours.

In investigating the action of corrosive poisons, it is a point of essential importance to ascertain, how much of their apparent effect is owing to chemical process, and how much is to be attributed to vital reaction. For this end, it is necessary in the first place to examine the bodies of animals immediately after death; and *secondly*, to discover what effect the poison has on dead animal matter.

Effect on dead Animal Matter.

A portion of the healthy stomach of a dog was held two minutes in a saturated solution, at 130° F., (such as they injected into the stomach.) The epidermis had been separated in a single flake, thickened and brittle, of a grayish colour, and upon the whole similar to what they have seen in the living stomach. The corion was translucent, its surface very pulpy, and the serous membrane was gray and crisped. When the immersion was prolonged five minutes, the whole corion became gelatinous.

They have likewise tried the effect of a saturated solution, at 50° F. In twenty hours, the villous coat was of a pale greenish-white colour and less adherent, but it was strong and its porous structure quite entire. In two days and a half it was brittle, and easily scraped off, and the other tunics were softened, swollen and translucent. In twelve days, the whole membranes could be spread out with the fingers, and in thirty days, they were dissolved to a semi-diffluent mass, soluble (with the exception of a small quantity of flocculent matter) in tepid water, yielding flocculi at the temperature of 130° F., and precipitating with tannin after ebullition. The same experiment was repeated in the human stomach ; which appears to have a somewhat greater power of resisting the action of the acid.

This action is a peculiar one, at least the mineral acids act in a very different manner. Nitric acid, diluted with twelve parts of water, soon renders the whole tunics brittle, dense, and of a lemon-yellow colour, without dissolving them; sulphuric acid similarly diluted gives them a pale cineritious tint, corrugates them at first, and then softens them slightly; and no farther change is produced by either in fourteen days.

In order to discover on which of the animal principles the dissolving power of oxalic acid depends, experiments were made with albumen, gelatin and fibrin, as these three products enter into the composition of the membranes of the stomach. Albumen forms the chief part of the mucous epidermis, and probably of the serous coat; gelatin forms the whole of the mucous corion and a considerable portion of the cellular tissue; and fibrin constitutes the greater part of the muscular tunic.

From these experiments it appears, that oxalic acid, when concentrated, coagulates albumen, but has no effect upon it in other circumstances. It gives to pure fibrin a degree of elasticity and translucency greater than it naturally possesses, but without dissolving it, and it bleaches common muscle, and preserves it from putrefaction, without sensibly altering its condition; but on the contrary, it dissolves gelatin, and even very rapidly.

When 25 grains of isinglass were placed in half an ounce of a temperate solution, containing 30 grains of the acid, it began to soften and swell in two or three minutes, and in twelve or sixteen hours was reduced to a uniform jelly-like mass. Pure water, at the same temperature, produced in thirty hours no other effect than slight softening and flexibility, but no solution, nor even viscosity of the surface.

This action is one of pure solution, in which neither body loses its characteristic proprieties; for though the proportion of gelatin be made exceedingly minute, the mixture has a tendency to gelatinize and precipitates with tannin; while on the other hand, how small soever be the proportion of acid, the mixture always reddens litmus.

Experiment 2d.

The *first* experiment with the *concentrated* acid was repeated upon another dog, under circumstances precisely the same, except that, half an hour before the poison was injected, they *removed an inch of the conjoined parvagum and sympathetic* on each side of the neck. The former animal we have seen, began to make violent efforts to vomit in two minutes, and died in twenty-one minutes. This dog, on the contrary, never had the slightest tendency to vomit. He soon became very restless, however, and in forty minutes, he was affected with irregularity in the fulness and quickness of breathing, slight tremor in the thoracic muscles, felt only by the hand, and peculiar dulness of sensation. In two hours and a half he began to stagger a little, but remained quite sensible : and three hours afterwards, was found in the agonies of death. This experiment was repeated several times and always gave analogous results.

It appears, therefore, that the division of the nerves connecting the stomach with the brain impedes very much the action of the concentrated acid. Death was caused in this case by absorption.

Experiments 3d and 4th.

Having thus ascertained its action, when highly concentrated, our next object was to discover whether, like the irritant poisons in general, its deleterious properties are impaired or destroyed by dilution.

With this view we gave to a dog, betwixt eight and ten pounds in weight, thirty-three grains of the concrete acid dissolved in six ounces, or eighty-seven parts of tepid water. In two minutes he made violent efforts to vomit; in eight and a half, he was seized with certain remarkable symptoms, (to be noticed afterwards,) very different from those detailed in the former experiments, and which we have universally found oxalic acid to produce, when much diluted. In half an hour from the beginning of the experiment he expired.

To place the distinction in a clearer point of view, the same quantity dissolved in two parts of tepid water, was therefore given to a dog of the same weight, and about the same age. In seven minutes he strove to vomit, and continued to do so at distant intervals, for an hour and a quarter. At that time the peculiar symptoms of this kind of poisoning began, and he died at the end of the sixth hour. It hence appears that *a small quantity of the acid kills an animal ten or twelve times sooner than when highly concentrated.*

Experiment 5th and 6th.

Into the stomach of two strong rabbits, of the same size and age, we injected a drachm of the acid, dissolved in eleven parts of lukewarm water. In one, the conjoined parvagum and sympathetic nerve were divided on each side of the neck; in the other they were left untouched. The latter in 8½ minutes began to breathe hurriedly, and to pull his head backwards on the spine. At the end of 10 minutes it was seized with paroxysms of most violent opisthotonos, and death took place 13 minutes after the commencement of the injection. In the former, whose nerves were previously divided, the breathing became hurried, and the head was thrown back 10 minutes after the injection began. In no long time it was attacked with violent opisthotonos, and in 14 minutes death was complete.

The three next experiments show its comparative effects when introduced by the stomach, by the pleura, and by the cellular tissue.

Experiment 7th.

Thirty-three grains dissolved in six drachms of water were injected into the stomach of a dog, weighing 18 to 20 pounds.

12*m.* Efforts to vomit, at distant intervals, and not very violent.

32*m.* Efforts rare; he hangs the head; the respiration is smooth, deep, regular, and not quickened.

47*m.* The efforts to vomit have ceased; the breathing continues the same; he walks sluggishly, and looks dull, but is perfectly sensible.

1*h.* 25*m.* He is affected with a peculiar kind of somnolency. He sits with his head drooping much, apparently unconscious of anything that goes on around him; yet he yelps when laid hold of, and is, in every respect, perfectly sensible. He breathes very smoothly and deeply. The pulsations of the heart are rather frequent and feeble. He staggers when forced to walk.

2h. 40m. Does not stagger so much. No other change.

4h. He is more feeble, but does not stagger, and is perfectly sensible.

24h. Some dulness, but he is quite sensible; and, except weakness, has no decided affection.

48h. Is both sensible and active, runs briskly about, and chews morsels of bread.

3 *days.* He was found lying on his side, nearly insensible, and breathing short and slow. When shaken, and put upon his legs, he tries to walk, but staggers and leans on the wall. The hind legs are very feeble.

3 *days.* 8*m.* Found dead. The body was examined 40 hours afterwards. The stomach was perfectly natural. There was no vascularity externally; and the internal membrane was quite entire, strong and white. The wound in the neck had sloughed and suppurated.

Experiment 8th.

The same quantity, similarly dissolved, was injected into the left pleura of a dog of about the same size. He struggled violently, and when let loose, ran to the other end of the room, apparently sensible, though dull.

10m. The breathing suddenly became hurried and very deep, both in inspiration and expiration. He hung his head, and though sensible, would not stir when struck. In a short while his tail was reversed, the respiration became very difficult, and almost suspended, and sank gradually down upon the belly; the breathing then became easier for a few seconds.

11m. Another paroxysm of suspended respiration, during which the tail was still more distinctly reversed, and the whole body spasmodically extended. Then, at

12m. the spasm relaxed, the whole body became

flaccid, and two or three convulsive gasps ensued at remote intervals.

The body was examined two days after death. The *pleura* was quite natural on both sides. Some blood, extravasated around the incision, was completely charred. There was a quantity of dirty, brownish-red semi-fluid matter in both sacs, rather sweet to the taste, and reddening litmus. The lungs were here and there scarlet on their surface, and gorged posteriorly. The villous coat of the stomach had a brownish-yellow tint at its œsophageal end, and there was lined with bile, but at the pyloric end was rosy-red and without bile. The whole intestines were natural internally and externally. The moisture of the peritoneum did not redden litmus.

Experiment 9th.

One hundred and sixty grains, dissolved in four cunces of water, were injected into the cellular tissue of a dog, weighing about thirty pounds, by a wound at the flexure of each thigh. The syringe was thrust three inches under the integuments; and when the injection was completed the wounds were carefully stitched, so that not a drop could escape. The fluid was felt forming different tumours on the lower part of the abdomen, and on the inside of each thigh.

13*m*. From the commencement of the injection he had some weakness and stiffness of the hind legs, and began to look dull.

45*m*. The hind legs are scarcely sensible when pricked, but the sensation of the rest of the body is unimpaired; the breathing is deep; he lies on his side.

50*m*. He rose with peculiar stiffness, and laid down again upon the belly, with the hind legs stretched out on one side, and the fore legs on the other; the hind legs are always stiff, and sometimes convulsively extended.

1h. 15m. The breathing became suddenly hurried. Soon afterwards there was some stiffness of the chest and neck. When raised, he stands stiffly in the same posture for a few seconds, and then sinks gently down upon the belly. He whines at intervals.

1h. 55m. He is much duller, but in other respects seemed to be improving till now, when the breathing again became suddenly hurried. The heart beats with great rapidity, and with such violence as to be heard at a short distance, all the limbs are rigid, and the neck slightly so. Though very dull, he continues quite sensible, for he shuts his eyelids if the hand is waved before him, and he follows a basin of water carried up and down.

2h. 12m. The breathing is still exceedingly hurried, but at times suspended for a few seconds; the heart still beats with extraordinary force; his dulness increases; he continues to walk about a little, but very stiffly; the tail has been gradually becoming stiff and straight.

2h. 20m. The suspension of breathing is more decided, now evidently depending upon spasms of the thoracic muscles, and is accompanied with reversion of the tail. These paroxysms cause him great agony, and they became gradually longer and more violent. Even in the intervals, the breathing is difficult and expiration convulsive.

2h. 45m. The pulsations of the heart are much more feeble, but still very frequent. The paroxysms of suspended respiration abate in violence, but the intervals are shorter.

2h. 55m. The paroxysms have ceased. The whole body is relaxed and in a state of complete coma; breathing short, frequent, and somewhat convulsive.

3h. 30m. No change, except that the breathing is slower and shorter.

4h. Breathing very short and only 14 in a minute; the pulsations of the heart cannot be felt.

14h. Found dead, cold and rigid.

The body was examined about 36 hours afterwards.

The muscles of the belly as high as the umbilicus, and the superficial muscles on the inside of each thigh, were pale, greenish and acid; but no fluid could be detected around them. The lungs were every where scarlet on their anterior surface, bluish-black posteriorly, scarlet internally; yet their air cells natural. The blood of the vena cava and aorta was dark, and very imperfectly coagulated; there was nothing unusual on the inside of the vessels. (In another case of the same kind the blood in the heart and the exhalations of all the serous surfaces, and the frothy fluid of the bronchi did not redden litmus.) The villous coat of the stomach was lined with bile, and stained brownish yellow. The rectum was redder than usual, not vascular, and the rest of the intestines perfectly healthy.

The next experiment shows the action of the poison when introduced at once into the veins.

Experiment 10th.

Eight grains and a half of acid were dissolved in 15 drachms of water at 100°, and 3 drachms slowly injected every five minutes, into the right femoral vein of a dog weighing about 20 pounds,—the inferior division of the vessel having been previously tied.

After the two first injections, the animal trembled, and the breathing became somewhat fuller; after the third, the breathing was slightly convulsive, but soon became again natural; thirty seconds after the fifth, he made a few sudden deep inspirations for half a minute, then some unavailing efforts to inspire, and died without a struggle. The heart did not pulsate after the last inspiration. (During a repetition of this experiment, the pulsations of the heart were observed to become suddenly very feeble, after each injection.) The body was then opened immediately. The right cavities of the heart were distended and not contractile. The blood in those cavities was dark, and had begun to coagulate; that in the left side was florid, fluid, and soon coagulated in the usual way. The blood in both these cavities did not redden litmus; and the serum, which had separated next day from that in the right side, gave no precipitate with hydrochlorate of lime. [Neither did that of the vena cava in another dog killed in the same manner.] The *muscles* preserved their contractility.

The two next experiments show the action of the poison introduced into the intestines, and the effect of applying it to a part, of which all connection with the body has been destroyed, except by blood-vessels.

Experiment 11*th*.

In a puppy of about eight or ten pounds weight, an ounce of water, containing 45 grains of acid, and at the temperature of 100°, was injected into a loop of small intestine two feet long; a single ligature was applied strongly at one end, and a double one at that by which the syringe was introduced.

19*m*. An attack of vomiting, preceded for some minutes by deep breathing, which afterwards became easier.

40*m*. Breathing small and frequent,—occasionally fuller, and somewhat convulsive; dulness.

1*h*. 18*m*. Breathing occasionally interrupted by a slight sudden expiration, like a short cough. Hind legs stiff. He hangs the head, and remains in the same posture.

1*h*. 45*m*. The breathing is quicker. The catches in expiration now occur together in paroxysms, and cause agony. Hind legs very rigid. Two slight extensions of the head and tail; posture very peculiar.

1*h*. 55*m*. There are now distinct spasmodic paroxysms. First, the breathing becomes convulsive, and deeper and deeper; at last, the chest is so firmly fixed, that with great effort he expands and contracts it only to a very small extent. Then the spasms relax, with gurgling cries and slight barking, and he soon breathes freely, but hurriedly. The legs are quite insensible.

2h. At the height of the paroxysm the breathing is wholly suspended.

2h. 35*m.* The paroxysms have become milder, he cannot stand when raised.

3*h.* Paroxysms less distinct, but longer, and accompanied with slight reversion of head and tail. Breathing in the intervals short; the eyes alone aré sensible.

3½*h.* He is now in a state of almost pure coma, without spasmodic paroxysms.

6*h.* Breathing slower and uniform, and expiration accompanied with a bark. Slight opisthotonos produced by touching his back smartly; but he has no other sign of sensation.

9*h.* Barking very feeble, no other change.

16*h.* Found dead and rigid.

The body was examined eight hours afterwards. The blood was equally dark in both systems. The intestines were perfectly natural, internally as well as externally. The ligatures were firm; most of the injected fluid gone. The fluid of the thoracic duct does not redden litmus.

Experiment 12*th.*

The last experiment was repeated on a puppy of the same size. But before the acid was injected, a double ligature was tied at each end of the portion of intestine, the gut divided betwixt them, and all its connections, by means of the mesentery, were then dissected away with great care, except four arteries and veins; the knife being carried round close to each vessel.

10*m.* Some stiffness of the hind legs. Begins to hang the head and look dull.

26*m.* An attack of vomiting, preceded, as in the last case, by deep respiration.

33*m.* The head and tail were twice extended slightly; breathing at times convulsive in expiration. Much duller.

1*h*. 7*m*. He is affected with a peculiar kind of dulness of sensation, or somnolency; will not rise, yet when raised, can both walk and stand. Expiration still convulsive.

1*h*. 30*m*. He is affected with paroxysms of suspended respiration, precisely as the other was in 1*h*. 55*m*.

2*h*. 5*m*. The paroxysms are now very distinctly marked, and are accompanied with more general tetanus than in the last animal. The insensibility has already become almost complete.

2*h*. 40*m*. The paroxysms of spasm have gradually and almost entirely subsided, and he now lies in a state of pure coma.

5*h*. 16*m*. He was found dead, warm and stiff. The body was opened seventeen hours afterwards. The ligatures were firm, and most of the injected fluid was gone. The mucous coat of the insulated portion of the intestine was somewhat softened, but not discoloured. There was no vascularity in any part of the intestines. The blood was black in both systems of vessels. The lungs were of a scarlet colour on many parts of their anterior surface.

Experiment 13*th*.

This experiment shows the action of the poison, when introduced into the sac of the peritoneum.

Twenty-two grains dissolved in four ounces of water were injected into the peritoneal sac of a strong cat, through an incision of the upper and lateral part of the abdomen; and the aperture was immediately secured with great care by stitches. Little pain seemed to follow the injection. The animal in a short while, however, began to be very restless and uneasy, and tried to vomit.

10*m*. It looked very dull, and twice jerked its head backwards.

11*m*. The heart beats feebly. It stretched out the

paws, and yawned; the tail became stiff; and the eyes nearly insensible.

12*m*. He now had general stiffness of the whole trunk and extremities, and made fruitless efforts to inspire.

13*m*. These were suddenly succeeded by relaxation of the whole body, and then by a few convulsive gasps and twitches of the lumbar muscles.

14*m*. The heart continued to tremble.

The body was examined 24 hours after death. The sac of the peritoneum contained scarcely a drachm of fluid, which reddened litmus. [In the case of another dog, twelve pounds in weight, that survived above nine hours, when 17 grains were injected into the peritoneum, we found nearly as much fluid as was introduced; but by analysis it was found to contain no acid, and to be, in fact, pure limpid serum; the peritoneum was also very vascular.] The peritoneum had a faint greyish-brown colour. The blood of the meseraic veins does not affect litmus. The stomach and intestines are natural internally. There are some irregular scarlet patches on the surface of the lungs.

From the foregoing experiments MM. Christison and Coindet infer, that oxalic acid acts by means of absorption. By the agency of the lungs the poison is decomposed, and its elements form with the principles of the blood, peculiar compounds to which the symptoms of poisoning are to be referred. And whatsoever, they add, may be the import of these speculations, they furnish ground enough for toxicologists to enter on a field of inquiry wholly new, yet probably rich in interesting results, viz.: what share have the lungs in the decomposition of poisons, that have been absorbed and mingled with the blood?

*Pommer** has published an account of the following experiments:

Five grains of oxalic acid dissolved in water, were

* Salzburger Medic. Chirurg. Zeitung. 1828, vol. ii. p. 203.

injected into the jugular vein of a spaniel. Eight seconds afterwards he breathed deeply, urinated, stretched his legs, and died. The heart's motion continued yet for 12 minutes, feeble and trembling; the blood did not act on litmus, and showed no vestige of oxalic acid; the lungs were healthy.

In a space of four minutes, at four separate times, 15 grains of oxalic acid were injected into the jugular vein of a dog. During the first injection the animal moaned; at the fourth it had spasms, stretched its legs, breathed twice profoundly, and was dead in half a minute. The motion of the heart was quickly extinguished; the blood was healthy, and showed no sign of acidity, nor of oxalic acid.

One grain of oxalic acid in 20 drops of water was injected into the jugular vein of a rabbit; it immediately stretched its feet, moved the forelegs convulsively, drew a deep breath, and died in half a minute. The heart was devoid of contractility.

Only when large quantities of oxalic acid were injected, did the blood redden litmus in the nearest vessels.

Fifteen grains of oxalic acid were injected into the abdominal cavity of a Pommeranian dog. During the process of injection he became slightly convulsed, and stretched out his forelegs. After four minutes he choked and then vomited, and in 10 minutes his gait became unsteady; he laid down; in 14 minutes he bent back the head, and became prostrate without showing any signs of sensibility or power of motion; the pulsation of the heart could not be observed; his breathing was short and deep, the mouth open, the pupils dilated; after 18 minutes he expired. The contractility of the intestines was gone; the blood of the lower vena cava, as well as that of the aorta was natural, not acid; the lungs sound. The right heart was yet contractile for 9 minutes. The epiploon was externally brownish, the surface of the intestines greyish, reddening litmus; most of the mesenteric veins contained brownish blood, which proved acid on testing.

Rave and Klosterman,* instituted among others the following experiments.

The œsophagus of a dutch mastiff, weighing ten pounds was opened, and a solution of 25 grains of oxalic acid in an ounce of distilled water, heated to 35° R., injected into the stomach by means of an elastic tube, and afterwards a ligature applied. In three minutes the animal began to howl, laid on his abdomen, and creeped over the room. In nineteen minutes he retched and made strong efforts to vomit, which only ceased a quarter of an hour before his death. The breathing became quick and troubled, the beatings of the heart very rapid. In half an hour the hind feet sank down paralysed, retaining, however, their sensibility; the head then fell down to the ground, moving from one side to the other. In three-quarters of an hour the dog became prostrate, and in two minutes more he died without convulsions, after having urinated considerably. He was immediately opened. The wound was of a dirty black colour, as if touched by lunar caustic. The interior of the chest unchanged; the heart was not contractile; the œsophagus inviolate, and on the exterior surface of the stomach and intestines no change; the contents of the first consisted partly of a brownish black fluid, in which swam flakes of the same colour, and which tasted sourish bitter, was inodorous, and did not change the colour of turmeric, partly of a brownish grey foam.

A 35° R. warm solution of twelve grains oxalic acid and six drachms of distilled water were injected through the anus into the intestines of a bitch, weighing over seven pounds, and the anus tied by a ligature. After the lapse of ten minutes a strong inclination for evacuation ensued, which, within twenty minutes increased to such a degree, that the animal effected a forcible passage through the ligature, and discharged some blackish fluid in small quantities. In half an hour a general tremor of

* Harless Jahrbuecher der deutschen, Medic. u. Chir. 2d. Supplt. Vol. 1827, p. 177.

the whole body took place, coming on by paroxysms. After that she vomited; the ejected matter consisted of half digested food. At the eighth hour the ligature was severed. During the night she discharged per anum a blackish very offensive fæces, mixed with streaks of blood. In it was discovered a worm one foot long, (tænia canina, *Pallas.*) The food, which was placed before her she did not touch, but drank freely and eagerly of cold water. Twenty-two hours from the commencement of the experiment she became very weak; put on her legs, she fell down again immediately. Some hours afterwards she fell into an asphytic sleep, in which she expired.

To a dog weighing eleven pounds, a small opening was made on the linea alba, near the navel, into which was injected a solution, 35° R., of sixteen grains of oxalic acid, mixed with four drachms of distilled water. The opening was closed by a ligature. Immediately after the injection the dog became very restless, jumped about and whined. In thirty-five minutes after passing his water and fæces, he vomited; the ejected matter was slimy, of a greenish colour, covered with a whitish foam. Soon after there appeared a tremor of the whole body, and the breathing became more rapid, and difficult. In six hours from the commencement of the experiment, he fell prostrate, stretched out his legs, and his eyes became fixed. Calls and pinching ceased to make any impression. He lay there for three-quarters of an hour, breathing slowly. The pulsation of the heart was also less. Shortly after he became convulsed and died.

Three grains of oxalic acid, mixed with three drachms of distilled water were injected into the same region near the navel of a rabbit, aged three months. During the first three minutes the animal moved about as usual; but soon after, it stretched itself down, and moved forward on the abdomen, making use only of the fore legs, for the hind legs seemed to be completely paralysed. Together with these symptoms, the breathing and beating of the heart became quicker. In nine minutes there appeared convulsions of all kinds, whilst the abdomen was inflated and very hard to the touch, the eyes became fixed, breathing slower. In this manner it remained for three minutes longer, after which it died in convulsions.

PATHOLOGICAL ANATOMY.

1. *In Animals.*—When an animal is examined immediately after death, no appearance of note is found in the brain, peritoneal sac or intestine. Unless death has been very rapid, the lungs are almost always studded on their surface with bright scarlet spots, and sometimes we have seen even the whole parenchyma of a uniform and beautiful scarlet colour. At the same time there never was any effusion, either in the air cells, or into their cellular tissue. In cases of poisoning that prove fatal before the stage of insensibility comes on, the heart, two or three minutes after death, is found neither contracting nor contractile; its pulmonary cavities are distended, and the blood is dark in those cavities and florid in the aorta. This fact is conformable with what we have observed in the same animals, first, at the time of death, viz: the contractions of the heart are almost imperceptible, even before the breathing ceases, and never continue after it. In the slowest cases, in which coma prevails for some time before death, the heart, though very feeble in its contractions towards the close, beats a little after the breathing has ceased, and then the blood is found equally dark in both vascular systems.

There is likewise an intermediate variety of poisoning wherein the stage of insensibility is short, and the heart scarcely survives the stoppage of respiration; and in such cases, the blood in the aortal cavities is darker than natural, but still considerably more florid than that of the veins and pulmonary cavities. (*Christison and Coindet.*)

Rave and Klosterman, after washing off the internal coat of the stomach, saw many dark brown spots, extending from the cardiac orifice, where they were most numerous, along the great curvature to within half an inch of the pyloric orifice. The spots formed longitudinal streaks, which always occupied the back part of the folds of the internal tunica. The interstices between these folds were either unchanged, or only coloured light yellow. The corroded cuticle was easily detached. The spots themselves, carefully scraped off, showed many small blood vessels. One and a half inch round the pyloric orifice, the internal cuticle was coloured yellow; the nearer the pylorus, the more the colouring decreased. In the duodenum and other intestines no changes were visible.

The bladder was distended with urine, and the kidneys, on making an incision, discharged large quantities of urine. In other cases the internal coat of the small intestines was reddened. In other respects the appearances were the same as those observed by Drs. *Christison* and *Coindet*.

2. *In Man.*—The examinations of dead bodies are both very deficient, and exceedingly discordant. The authors, generally, were neither sufficiently precise in their phraseology, nor minute in their descriptions. A reddish froth sometimes issues from the mouth and nose. In one case there was a good deal of general emphysema, ten hours after death.

The brain has been rarely examined. In one case the cerebral organs were turgid; in another case there was some effusion under the arachnoid, appearances probably independent of disease.

In the three best described cases, the appearance of throat and stomach, etc., was the following.

1st. The mucous coat of the throat and gullet looked as if it had been scalded, and that of the gullet could be easily scraped off. The stomach contained a pint of thick fluid. This is usually dark, like coffee grounds, as it contains a good deal of blood. The inner coat of the stomach was pulpy, in many parts black, in others red. The inner membrane of the intestines was similarly, but less violently affected. The outer coat of both stomach and intestines was inflamed. The lining membrane of the windpipe was also very red. (*Hebb.*)

2d. The inside of the gullet was pale, as if boiled, strongly corrugated, and brittle, and covering a ramification of vessels filled with consolidated blood. The stomach presented externally numerous vessels in the same state, and its villous coat was pale, soft, and brittle, but here and there injected with vessels. The duodenum, and part of the jejunum, were red; the other intestines natural; the liver, spleen and kidneys congested. The stomach contained a brownish jelly, in which gelatine was detected, as well as oxalic acid. The blood was fluid every where, except in the vessels of the gullet and stomach.

3d. The whole villous coat of the stomach was either softened or removed, as well as the inner membrane of the gullet, so that the muscular coat was exposed; and this coat presented a dark gangrenous-like appearance, being much thickened and highly injected.

These are the most common signs of its action, but cases have occurred where no such signs of violent irritation have been observed. In the case of a girl, who died about thirty minutes after swallowing an ounce of the acid, no morbid appearance whatsoever was to be seen, in any part of the alimentary canal. In the case of another girl, where death took place in twenty minutes, there was no appearance but contraction of the rugæ of the gullet and stomach, one spot of extravasation on the latter, and doubtful softening of the villous coat.*

Dr. John Mollan, in the case of poisoning related by him in the Dublin Hospital Reports says, "one circumstance deserves notice from its infrequency, namely, the discovery of air in the right cavities of the heart. I am not aware that any thing similar has been observed in

* Christison on Poisons.

cases of sudden death, produced by any deleterious substance, and I am at a loss to account for its production."

In one case communicated in October, 1844, by Dr. H. Letheby, in the London Lancet, the tissue of the stomach was so softened and disorganized, that it could scarcely be handled without tearing. At the cardiac end it was reduced to a soft, pulpy, gelatinous substance, and had numerous perforations in consequence. The contents which had been saved in a glass amounted to about six ounces in quantity; they had a very dark colour resembling porter. On being tested they were found to contain about three drachms of oxalic acid.

Antidotes,—(when taken in large doses.) As the vomiting in such cases is speedy and continual; emetics are unnecessary and will often fail of their effect; besides during the time lost before their operation, the acid would in general have acted long enough to prove fatal. Vomiting may be promoted by tickling the throat. Mr. Thompson found, that large quantities of chalk, given after the dangerous symptoms had begun, speedily removed them, and restored the animals to health.* The results of his experiments have been applied to poisoning in man, and in one of the cases of recovery the antidote was used with advantage. Its effect is evidently owing to the insolubility of the oxalate of lime. Magnesia has also been advantageously given. The reporter observes that the first dose was followed by instantaneous relief from the burning pain in the stomach. According to Dr. Christison it is the best of all chemical antidotes, and preferable to carbonate of lime, which occasions considerable inconvenience on account of the sudden extrication of a large quantity of carbonic acid gas. Yet chalk will be oftener employed, since it is more frequently at hand, and there is no room for delay in the selection of remedies.

In the two cases of recovery recorded, small doses of opium were administered after the use of chalk and

*Med. Rep. Vol. iii., Thomson's Experiments.

magnesia, and the vomiting soon became less violent. One of them took brandy with advantage, and the other experienced much relief from friction and hot fomentations. Drs. Christison and Coindet also recommend ammonia and ether, as worthy of trial. The stomach pump may be used, but on account of the rapidity with which this poison acts, it is not advisable to lose time by its application, until after the antidote has been administered.

LEGAL MEDICINE.

The cases hitherto published have been the result of accident, and happened chiefly in London from the carelessness of apothecaries. Several cases have, however, also occurred in Germany.

Oxalic acid has been hitherto given through accident only. There is reason to fear, that, when its properties are more generally known, it may also be given by design. Much inducement is already held out to the poisoner by the readiness with which it may be administered; and it will be no small additional temptation, that, in certain circumstances, there will be as much difficulty in detecting it.

The medical evidence will be derived, as in the case of other poisons,—first, from the symptoms; second, from the morbid appearances; and, third, from the chemical analysis of the contents of the stomach and intestines, of the coats of the stomach, of the vomited matters, and of suspected articles of food.

1. The symptoms can rarely lead to more than a suspicion of general poisoning. Yet, burning pain of the stomach after taking a medicine, speedy, violent and incessant vomiting, followed by loss of the pulse, convulsions, insensibility, and death within an hour, are symptoms of no natural disease, and are caused conjunctly by no poison, except oxalic acid.

2. A general or partial abrasion of the mucous epi-

dermis, *gelatinization and translucency of the corion*, or even of the other coat, and charring of the blood in their vessels, might be decisive of the cause of death. But as in these cases the acid will always be found, it should be sought for.

All the other morbid appearances are unsatisfactory.

3. *Analysis of the suspected matters.*—The stomach is to be washed with pure water, and if disorganized, preserved for analysis. The washings, the contents of the stomach, the vomited matter, and the disorganized tissues and suspected articles of food are to be boiled separately, a little pure water being added if necessary. If chalk or magnesia has been used as an antidote, what remains on the filter, (except that from the tissues,) is to be preserved for analysis. The filtered fluid is to be tried first with litmus paper, and then by the three following tests—the hydrochlorate of lime, the sulphate of copper, and the nitrate of silver.

1st. Decolourize the fluid, if necessary, with chlorine. The hydrochlorate of lime, dropped into a solution containing oxalic acid, or an oxalate, especially the latter, throws down an insoluble oxalate of lime. But it also precipitates with the carbonates, sulphates, phosphates, tartrates, citrates, and with all their acids, but the carbonic. The following mode of procedure will serve to distinguish it from these substances. The nitric acid will not take up the sulphate of lime, but a few drops of it dissolve the oxalate. The hydrochloric acid will not dissolve the oxalate, unless added in very large quantity, while two or three drops will take up the carbonate, phosphate, tartrate or citrate.

2d. Decolourize a second portion of the fluid with chlorine. The sulphate of copper precipitates oxalic acid bluish-white, and the oxalates pale blue. This test is sufficiently delicate and useful, since the sulphate of copper does not affect fluids that contain sulphuric, hydrochloric, nitric, tartaric, citric acids, or their ordinary salts. It precipitates the carbonates, and throws down phosphoric acid, whether free or combined. The oxalate, however, is easily distinguished; for it is insoluble in hydrochloric acid, while a few drops of that acid at once take up the phosphate or carbonate.

3d. The nitrate of silver produces a heavy white precipitate with oxalic acid, and still better with the oxalates; and this precipitate, when dried and heated over a candle, becomes brown on the edge, then of a sudden fulminates faintly, and is all dispersed in white fumes. When impure, it deflagrates like gun powder, and when in too small quantity to be collected, the filtering paper burns, as if steeped in nitrate of potash. This is a very characteristic and delicate test.

From a quarter of a grain of oxalic acid, dissolved in 4000 parts of water, we have procured enough of the powder to show its fulmination twice. The precipitation alone cannot be trusted to, for it may equally take place with hydrochloric, phosphoric, citric or tartaric acid, and likewise with the alkalies. But when the test of fulmination is tried, there is no chance of its being confounded with any of these, except perhaps with the tartaric and citric acid. The compounds of these acids with silver, we find, possess properties that will render the nitrate of silver one of the simplest and most correct tests for distinguishing them from each other, and from oxalic acid. The citrate of silver becomes brown under exposure to heat, froths up, then deflagrates slightly, with the discharge of white fumes, and a large quantity of dull, ash-grey, crumbling matter remains, of a very peculiar fibrous structure. The tartrate of silver becomes brown, froths up like the citrate, white fumes are discharged, without even deflagration, and there is left an ash coloured botryoidal mass, incrusted outwardly with silver.

If magnesia or chalk has been given as an antidote during the patient's life, the oxalate of magnesia or lime may be mingled, in the form of powder, with the contents of the stomach; or with the vomited matter. The powdery matter is then to be separated by elutriation from what remains upon the filter during the previous process. If magnesia has been the antidote employed, it is only requisite to boil the powder in pure water for a few minutes, and then subject the filtered fluid to the three tests described above. For the oxalate of that earth is sufficiently soluble to furnish, even with a single ounce of water, a solution in which all the foregoing characters may be observed. If the antidote employed has been chalk, then the powder is to be boiled for fifteen minutes with half its weight of pure subcarbonate of potash, dissolved in 20 to 30 parts of water. A mutual interchange then takes place, and the solution contains oxalate and carbonate of potash. In applying the tests to this solution, the free alkali is to be previously neutralized with hydrochloric acid, when hydrochlorate of lime or sulphate of copper is to be used, and with nitric acid, before using the nitrate of silver. In the last case there ought to be as little excess of acid as possible, because the oxalate of silver is soluble in nitric acid.

These tests of oxalic acid are very little influenced by the presence of such animal matter as may exist in the suspected fluid after boiling and filtration. The chief animal principle then present is gelatin. Gelatin alone is not precipitated by hydrochlorate of lime, sulphate of copper, or nitrate of silver; neither does it affect the delicacy of the two first as tests of oxalic acid; but when in very large proportion, it suspends the action of nitrate of silver. Whenever this obstacle is encountered, or if, from any other cause we have left unexamined, this the most decisive of the tests does not give satisfactory results, the oxalic acid may be thrown down with the hydrochlorate of lime, and the insoluble oxalate boiled with carbonate of potass as just described. This process will probably be always proper, when the suspected fluid is deeply coloured; for we cannot decolourize it with chlorine, since chlorine precipitates abundantly with that salt. (*Christison and Coindet.*)

GENERAL VIEW OF THE ACTION OF OXALIC ACID ON ANIMALS.

In giving a general view of the action of oxalic acid Drs. Christison and Coindet assert, that the symptoms differ according to the quantity given, and to the degree in which it has been diluted. They likewise differ somewhat according to the tissue to which it has been applied—and further, they vary in different species of animals. They are seen most characteristically when the acid has been so given as not to prove fatal for an hour or more.

If, with this view, a small quantity be injected into the stomach, intestines or peritoneum of a dog, he is soon seized with violent efforts to vomit. But the *first unequivocal sign* of its action is generally a *slight permanent stiffness* of *the hind legs*, drooping of the head, weakness, and *increased frequency of the pulse*, and a very peculiar dull, sorrowful look. About the same time there appears a slight sudden check in inspiration, from the respiratory muscles contracting before the chest is fully expanded. Gradually several of these come together, so as to constitute paroxysms of short hurried breathing, with intervals of ease. Meanwhile *the stiffness of the hind legs increases;* they become likewise *insensible*, and often the spasm gives place to *paralysis;* he jerks the head occasionally backwards, *walks with a peculiar stiff gait*, and assumes very odd postures, from inability to regulate the motions of the limbs. As the poisoning advances, the motions of the chest during the paroxysms become more and more confined by spasm of the muscles; and at last there is a period towards the close of each paroxysm, when the spasm is so great as completely to suspend the respiration. This is commonly accompanied with more or less extension of the head, tail and extremities, sometimes amounting to *violent opisthotonos*. In the intervals, the breathing continues hurried, and the heart beats very feebly and rapidly. In one case only we observed it prodigiously strong, so that it might be heard a few feet from the animal. The insensibility hitherto limited to the hind legs, now extends to the trunk and fore legs, and lastly the head. As the insensibility increases, the breathing diminishes in frequency, the spasmodic paroxysms become more and more obscure, and then cease altogether. For some time, however, they may be slightly renewed, by striking the back and limbs; but at last the animal falls into a state of deep pure coma, with complete relaxation of the whole body. The heart now can scarcely be felt; the breathing is slow, regular and short, and becomes gradually more obscure, till finally life is extinguished without a struggle.

Several striking variations are produced by differences in the dose. Thus, if it be augmented, the fits of spasm come on early and with great violence, the intervals are marked by remissions only, and the animal expires in a paroxysm, before the stage of insensibility begins. The action then resembles considerably that of the vegetable alkalies, brucia and strychnia, but differs from it in being also exerted, as we shall soon see, upon the heart. Death may be produced in this manner, in three, five or ten minutes.

If on the other hand, the dose be much diminished, there may be stiffness of the hind legs, much dulness, drooping of the whole body, and a sort of somnolency, without insensibility, or even without spasmodic paroxysms, and then the animal will commonly recover. In such cases, notwithstanding the local irritating power of the acid, inflammation is not apt to ensue. The diluted state is in part the cause of this.

Similar modifications arise *from the degree to which the acid is diluted; dilution having nearly the same effect as increase of quantity.**

The symptoms likewise vary somewhat, according to

* This remarkable observation is literally transcribed from Christison's and Coindet's interesting Memoir.

the tissue to which it is applied. Thus no vomiting precedes the spasmodic symptoms, if the poison has been injected into the pleura or cellular tissue. Moreover we have always found the paroxysms of spasm to be most remarkable, when it was applied to the serous tissues. Death ensues quickest when the acid is introduced directly into the veins.

Lastly they vary in different species of animals. Thus cats are more rapidly killed by it than rabbits inferior in size, and frequently the spasmodic paroxysms are not distinct. In *rabbits* the *opisthotonos* is always remarkably violent. When a drachm in twelve parts of water is introduced into the stomach, the trunk and extremities during the paroxysms are extended with such suddenness and force, that the whole body is often raised nearly two feet into the air.

The order of the symptoms and appearances after death seems to indicate, that the *primary action of the poison is on the spinal marrow and brain, and the heart and lungs are effected secondarily, through the injury done to the nervous system.*

Thus the first symptom observed is spasmodic contraction, or sometimes paralysis of the hind legs; next, the trunk is similarly effected, as is shown by the spasm of the muscles of respiration; and then the animal becomes insensible, which marks the commencement of an affection of the brain. The functions of the heart and lungs begin to suffer as soon as the insensibility begins, the pulsations of the heart becoming feeble and hurried, and the impeded respiration bringing on symptoms of incomplete asphyxia.

These two functions are variously affected in different circumstances. When the dose has been small, the heart suffers less; the signs of an injury of the brain are fully developed, and end in pure coma,—in consequence of which the animal dies slowly, asphyxiated. This is shown not only by the symptoms, but likewise by the heart contracting after death, and by the arterial system being filled with black blood. But when the dose has been greater, the heart's action is destroyed at once through a sudden impression conveyed from the origin of the nerves, before the symptoms either of coma or of asphyxia can be developed; for then the heart does not contract after death, and the blood in its aortal cavities is florid. It is a curious confirmation of this secondary action on the heart, that precisely the same appearances are found when the nervous system has been powerfully irritated, not through absorption, but by sympathy with extensive injury of the stomach. In that case, too, the heart loses its contractility as soon as the animal expires, and its aortal cavities contain florid blood. (*Christison and Coindet.*)

The experiments of Rave and Klosterman, as well as those of Pommer, completely confirm the above observations of Drs. Christison and Coindet. The experiments of Pommer, who used a still smaller quantity of the poison in his injections than Drs. Christison and Coindet, fully establish the fact, that in proportion to the diminution of the quantity and its dilution, if injected into a vein, the more rapidly death ensues. It is true, we have no data of the weight of the animals, which he used in his experiments. The injection of the poison into the jugular, instead of the femoral vein, as was done by Christison and Coindet, might also hasten death. But in whatever light we may view the experiments, there is no reason to doubt the truth of this proposition.

It is unnecessary for me to dwell here on the strong confirmation which the doctrines of the Homœopathic school may draw from the facts here proclaimed. But let those, who are in the habit of smiling at these doctrines, carefully examine and sift them. They will at least not be able to accuse Drs. Christison and Pommer of partiality.

THERAPEUTIC OBSERVATIONS.

Only few decided observations may be ventured upon the curative powers of oxalic acid. Most of the provers have taken it but once, and on the female organism it has not been tried at all, if I except one observation. Further experiments will be necessary to enlighten us about the whole range of its action on the healthy human body.

The observation of Drs. Christison and Coindet, that oxalic acid acts primarily on the brain, and secondarily, on the heart and lungs, seems also to be corroborated by the experiments upon the healthy human economy.

All provers seem to have felt its action first in the head, and afterwards in the heart and lungs. It has a most decided action on the vertex and forehead, and seems to produce in its secondary effect great exhilaration of spirits, with other peculiar effects upon the mind.

Its action on the abdomen in the region of the navel with colic and difficult emission of flatulency, is very decided. I have cured a chronic inflammation of the abdomen in the region of the navel, in the case of a child, æt. 5, with a few small doses of oxalic acid, where several other remedies had proved ineffectual.

Jaeggy speaks highly of it as an anti-phlogistic, in small fractional doses in most inflammations of the abdominal viscera, hepatitis and psoitis excepted.

Its effect on the urinary organs and testicles, is also prominent, although the experiments are too few in number to admit of the establishment of more direct indications for its choice in any particular case.

I have prescribed it with benefit in a case of chronic soreness and heaviness in the testicles, accompanied with a bruised sensation in the os sacrum, and general weakness of the genitals. There were also many symptoms indicating tabes dorsalis.

It will probably prove serviceable in laryngitis, diseases of the chest and heart, rheumatic affections of the joints, and also lameness of the lower extremities. A palpitation of the heart, occurring at night after lying down in bed, and depending on a rheumatic affection of the heart, was entirely cured by oxalic acid.

The assertion of *Valli*, that in oxalic acid we should probably find a remedy that would prolong life, seems to be merely theoretical. His theory is, that oxalic acid would have the effect of retaining the animal lime in a fluid form, and in a condition to be carried off, thereby preventing its becoming compact, and the brittleness of the solids, depending thereon, as well as the obstruction of the vessels. This theory, based entirely upon chemical laws, seems to lose complete sight of its powerful dynamical effect.

I have repeatedly prescribed the 2*d* and 3*d* trituration, to persons of different ages, with a view to the above effect, but without any visible operation. Whether by giving larger doses a different result might have been obtained, I am not prepared to say.

The following are the pathogenetic effects of the 1*st* and 2*d* trituration of oxalic acid. Those of Dr. Christison, are taken from cases of poisoning.

GENERAL SYMPTOMS.—1. All the pains from oxalic acid, seem to occupy only a small spot, half an inch to an inch in length, viz: in the eustachian tube, right wrist, right hypochondrium, region of navel, knee, etc. (*Hering.*)

They seem to be excited and aggravated by movement, as the pains in the bowels, testicles, kidney, back, etc. (*Neidhard.*)

From time to time he has those peculiar jerking pains, like short stitches, confined to a small spot, and lasting only a few seconds. (*Hering.*)

Oxalic acid has a decided action on the joints: ankle, knees, hips, wrist, shoulders. (*Neidhard.*)

5. Extreme lassitude of the body. (*Neidhard.*)

Pain, but chiefly great lassitude and weakness of the limbs, and next morning numbness, and weakness there as well as in the back. This affection was at first so severe, that she could hardly walk up stairs.

She recovered entirely in a few days. *Christison.* (In the case of a girl who had swallowed by mistake about two drachms.)

A feeling, as after a debauch the previous night; dull headache, with a gnawing, tensive pain and soreness in the eyes, and superciliary regions, lassitude, disinclination to occupation, reading, etc., and inclination to stretch, with occasional yawning. Relief by walking in the cool open air. (Next day, after taking oxalic acid. 2*d*. *Kitchen.*)

Tremor of the limbs. (Mitheilungen des Vereins fuer Natur und Heilkunde im voigtlaendischen Kreise.)

A very singular ease in his motions. (*Hering.*)

10. A peculiar general numbness, approaching to palsy. *Christison.*

Loss of consciousness for eight hours. *Christison.* (From two drachms.)

Nervous symptoms appear mostly in those patients, who have taken the diluted acid. *Christison.*

Convulsions either at the time of death or before it. *Christison.*

Convulsions, with two or three deep inspirations before death. *Christison.*

15. The symptoms from oxalic acid occasionally intermit for some hours or a day, and then return in a diminished degree. (*Neidhard.*)

Some, who are generally much affected by cold weather, appear better able to bear it. (*Neidhard.*)

SKIN.—During shaving, the skin is more sensitive. (*Hering.*)

The face is redder than usual. (*Hering.*)

Red points on the glans penis, without itching or any other sensation. (*Hering.*)

20. In the evening after walking, during sitting, a violent itching on a small spot of the neck, the right side of the hairy scalp, and on the left side of the trunk, etc. (*Hering.*)

Itching on the neck. (*Neidhard.*)

Smarting soreness around the neck, as if chafed by the collar. (*Williamson.*)

On a spot on the right index finger, where a cut from a penknife had healed four days ago, a very painful pustule appears. (From oxalic acid. 2*d*. *Neidhard.*)

An eruption or mottled appearance of the skin, in circular patches, not unlike the roundish red marks on the arms of stout healthy children, but of a deeper tint. *Christison.*

SLEEP.—25. Slept very little through the night, and when he did, had constant dreams with starting and then waking up with fright. The dreams were of an unpleasant character. (1st night. *Dubs.*)

He raised himself up in bed in alarm, looking round the room, but on recollecting where he was, he laid down again, repeating the same action in an hour. (1st night, from ox. ac. 3 grs. of $\frac{1}{10}$ trit. *Dubs.*)

Being awakened by a noise in the night, he could not go to sleep again for two hours. (*Floto.*)

Continual and vivid dreams, always of a frightful nature; he wakes up often and dreams constantly. (*Neidhard.*)

Sleep very restless, but without dreams. (2d day. *Neidhard.*)

30. Has had dreams, which he cannot remember. (First night. *Hering.*)

Very profound and long sleep; on rising from bed quite stupid, he lies down again and sleeps one hour longer. (2d day. *Hering.*)

Very violent yawning. (*Floto.*)

Great sleepiness in the morning. (2d day. *Hering.*)

After dinner, sleepiness, and profound sleep while in the sitting position. (*Neidhard.*)

35. He is more inclined to sleep at night than usual. (*Neidhard.*)

Dreams of rapidly sliding walking, he glides on his way with every step without difficulty; dreams also that water is poured upon him. (2d day. *Hering.*)

Dreams of an agreeable and lascivious nature, and of a character of reality. (*Kitchen.*)

FEVER.—Creeping of cold, particularly from the lower part of the spine upwards. (*Neidhard.*)

In the evening, after tea, sneezing, with chilliness. (*Neidhard.*)

An internal sensation of heat, particularly in the face, for several hours during the forenoon. (*Hering.*)

40. Some heat at first in the face, and afterwards in the left leg, like from external warmth. (*Hering.*)

General sensation of heat. (*Neidhard.*)

Exhausting fever with dyspepsia and singultus. *Christison.* (In a patient, who seemed at first to be doing well, but was carried off afterwards with the above fever in twenty-three days.)

Flushes of heat and perspiration all over the body. (*Dubs.*)

Clammy perspiration. *Christison.*

45. His hands, feet and face were cold and covered with a cold perspiration. (Mittheilungen, s. loc. cit.)

He perspires less than usual. (*Floto.*)

Pulse more frequent and harder than usual. (*Floto.*)

Pulse increased in frequency, from 100 to 108. (*Hering*, *Neidhard.*)

The pulse is more frequent than usual, and tense. (*Kitchen.*)

50. The pulse in every case became imperceptible, and even in those who recovered, it could not be felt for several hours. This state of the pulse was accompanied with deadly coldness, clammy sweats, sometimes lividity of the nails and fingers. *Christison.* (Contrary to this general fact, observes Dr. C., he once remarked in a dog the pulsation of the heart so strong, as to be audible at the distance of several yards.)

Extreme feebleness of the pulse. *Christison.* (From two scruples after 24 hours.)

Pulse small, tremulous, intermittent. (Mittheilungen, s. loc. cit.)

General excitement in the evening. (*Neidhard.*)

MENTAL.—In the morning, power of meditation

very difficult and slow ; is hardly able to answer questions proposed to him. (2d day. *Hering.*)

55. Disinclination to conversation. (*Floto.*)

Sensation of fulness in the face, and excitement, with disinclination to conversation. (1st day. *Hering.*)

Seems in its primary action to diminish the power of concentrating his ideas, and afterwards to increase it. (*Neidhard.*)

Unusual power of concentration of the mind. (*Williamson.*)

Greater presence of mind, the relations of the world seem to be clearer to him. (*Neidhard.*)

60. The pains from oxalic acid, as soon as *he thinks about them*, return, particularly that in the knee, the hiccup, etc. (*Hering.*)

Philoprogenitiveness, (?) greater love of his children, in one in whom this feeling was always predominating; a decidedly expressed, and clearly distinguishable symptom, it being not traceable to any other cause. (*Hering.*) Compare 74.

He feels more composed than usual, and very much exhilarated. (*Neidhard.*)

General exhilaration of the mind. (3d day. *Hering.*)

Hilarity and cheerfulness. (*Williamson.*)

65. Great cheerfulness of the mind, quicker in thought and action. (*Neidhard.*)

The whole forenoon unusual vivacity, and power of concentration, which is still more decided in the afternoon. (*Neidhard.*)

Great increase of animation through the day, with playfulness and mirthfulness, which has not of late years been natural to him. (1st, 2d, and 3d day. *Dubs.*)

Nervous and vascular excitement, as from alcohol, constituting a feeling of hilarity, and the pulse one-third more frequent than usual, and tense. (*Kitchen.*)

HEAD.—Giddiness the whole day. (*Neidhard.*)

70. On lying down vertigo, like a swimming towards the left side. (*Hering.*)

Emptiness in the head, sensation of faintiness, as if all the blood had left the brain, with anxiety. (*Floto.*)

Sensation in the upper part of the body, and particularly the head, as if the blood was streaming from below upwards, and from within outwards. (*Hering.*)

Headache. *Christison.* (24 hours after taking two scruples.)

Pain pressing inwardly between the vertex and occiput, on a spot not larger than a dollar, on the middle line. (In quarter of an hour. *Hering.*)

75. Pain along the base of the occipital bone, returning several times, during the first two days. (*Williamson.*)

In the morning after rest slight aching in the occiput, and erections. (*Hering.*)

Slight compression in the head, with a sensation like a screw behind each ear. (*Hering.*)

Soon after taking it, pain on the vertex. (*Floto.*)

Dull headache on the vertex. (From one-tenth ox. ac. *E. Smith.*)

80. Heaviness in the forehead and vertex. (In the morning, after taking the acid in the evening. *E. Smith.*)

Continual dull pain in the forehead and vertex. (*Dubs.*)

Flushes of heat and perspiration in the morning, with sharp pains in the forehead and vertex. (*Dubs.*)

Sharp pains in the forehead and vertex, with a feeling of lightness. The pain is most acute over the left eye, and in the left temple. (Soon after taking it. *Dubs.*)

Dull pains, with occasional sharp pains in the forehead. (*Dubs.*)

Dull headache. Compare 7.

85. Fulness in the forehead above the eyes. (*Neidhard.*)

Removes immediately a dulness in the forehead, to which he was frequently subject in the morning. (*Neidhard.*)

Painful pressure in the right temple, (confined to a small spot) the pain is also jerking, sliding; soon after, the same sensation in the hollow of the left knee. (*Hering.*)

Pain in the left temple, extending as far as the lower jaw. (In 1½ hours. *Neidhard.*)

Jerking in the left temple. (*Neidhard.*)

EYES.—90.—Pressure in the upper part of the eyes during walking. (*Floto.*)

Pain in both orbits, but worse in the left one. *Williamson.*)

Linear objects appear larger and more distant, than they really are. (In one who is near sighted. *Hering.*)

EARS.—In the afternoon occasionally a pain in the depth of the ear, as in if the eustachian tube, near the throat; worse on the right side. (*Hering.*)

A kind of slight blowing noise in the left ear. (*Neidhard.*)

NOSE.—95. Watery running from the nose, with sneezing. (*Floto.*)

Pain in the nose. (*Hering.*)

Sneezing with chilliness. Compare 38.

FACE, JAWS.—Sensation of fulness in the face. (*Hering.*)

An internal sensation of heat, particularly in the face. Compare 39.

Some heat at first in the face, and afterwards in the left leg. Compare 40.

The face is redder than usual. 18.

Drawing pain with rigidity near the angle of the lower jaw, first in the left, then in the right side, but longer in the left. (*Floto.*) Compare 88.

TEETH.—Dull aching pains of the molar teeth of the right and left upper jaw, worse in the right jaw. (Lasted nearly all day, but passed away towards evening. *Dubs.*)

100. Dull pain in the first molar tooth of the right upper jaw, which is very distressing. (After 15 minutes *Dubs.*)

Bleeding of the gums during friction of them. Has had the same occasionally before, but it was this time unexpectedly soon, and much more copious. (*Hering.*)

MOUTH.—Inflammation of the tongue and mouth, if the acid has had time to develop its operation. *Christison.*

The tongue was red, swollen, tense and tender, the day after the acid was swallowed. *Christison.*

Tongue dry, sore and excoriated, worse towards the point, continued all day and evening. (*Dubs.*)

105. The tongue felt rather more cool than hot. (Mittheilungen, s. loc. cit.)

In rincing the mouth, a *sour taste* in it. (1st day. *Hering.*)

In the forenoon a decidedly sour taste in the mouth. (2d day. *Hering.*)

THROAT.—Soreness of the fauces on swallowing, for two hours in the morning. (*Dubs.*) Compare 122.

* The chronic sore throat, to which he is subject, feels much better. (*Hering.*)

110. Expectoration of thick yellowish mucus from the throat. (*Floto.*)

Augments in the first hour the secretion of mucus from the throat. (*Neidhard.*)

STOMACH, APPETITE.—*Eructations of tasteless wind after each meal.* (*Dubs.*)

Eructations of wind, tasting of the food he has eaten. (*Dubs.*)

Eructations and discharge of flatulency per anum. (*Floto.*)

115. Eructations and passage of flatulency downwards. (*E. Smith.*)

Hiccup, which continues for some time, although he has taken nothing substantial. (1st day. *Hering.*) Compare 60.

Vomiting. *Christison.* (Only from very large doses.)

Slight sickness of the stomach. (*Neidhard.*)

Qualmishness of the stomach with sickness. (After 6 hours. *Neidhard.*)

120. A sensation of grasping in the stomach, very transient. (In a few seconds. *Neidhard.*)

Slight gnawing, burning in the stomach and eructations. (In 1½ hours. *Neidhard.*)

Burning pain in the stomach, and generally also in the throat. *Christison.* (Immediately in every case.*)

Pressure in the stomach. (In a few minutes. *Neidhard.*)

He wakes up at night with a most *violent pressive pain*, like a heavy weight in the pit of the stomach; it comes and goes at intervals of 15 minutes, but diminishes in force at each renewal. It lasts altogether about 2 hours. Discharge of flatulency relieves the pain. (After 5 drops of oxalic ether, taken in the morning. *Neidhard.*)

125. Severe pain in the stomach. *Christison.* (From seven drachms.)

Excruciating pain in the stomach. (Mittheilungen s. loc. cit.)

The slightest touch of the stomach caused the most violent pains. (Mittheilungen, s. l. c.)

Excessive sensibility of the stomach, with disposition to costiveness. (Mittheilungen, etc., in a patient who recovered, but who remained for a long time subject to those symptoms.)

His natural weakness of the stomach is much diminished. (2d day. *Neidhard.*)

130. In the evening after tea, pyrosis, with much emission of flatulency, and pressing downwards. (*Neidhard.*)

* Oxalic acid is one of the poisons, of whose operation distinct evidence may sometimes (though certainly not always) be found in the symptoms. If a person immediately after swallowing a solution of a crystalline salt, which tasted purely and strongly acid, is attacked with burning in the throat, then with burning in the stomach, vomiting, particularly of bloody matter, imperceptible pulse and excessive langour, and dies in half an hour, or still more in twenty, fifteen, or ten minutes, I do not know any fallacy which can interfere with the conclusion, that oxalic acid was the cause of death. No parallel disease begins so abruptly and terminates so soon; and no other crystalline poison has the same effect.—*Christison on Poisons.*

Every evening pyrosis. (*Neidhard.*)

Great increase of appetite. (*Hering.*)

Loss of appetite. (*Neidhard.*)

No thirst, and rather a repugnance to water. (*Dubs.*)

135. Unusual thirst at 3 o'clock, A. M. (2d day. *Neidhard.*)

Violent thirst. (Mittheilungen, etc.)

A sensation in the fauces, as if there was acidity in the stomach. (2d day. *Hering.*)

BOWELS.—Bowels opened in the morning, at 9 o'clock, and again at 4 in the afternoon. Slight colic pain in and around the umbilicus, just before the afternoon evacuation. (*Dubs.*)

Pain like a cramp a little to the left of the umbilicus, and several minutes after, colic pain in the right iliac region. Eructations of tasteless winds several times. (1st day. 5 o'clock, P. M. *Dubs.*)

140. Distressed feeling around the navel, and through the whole abdomen, with a sensation of great weakness in the latter. (2d day. *Dubs.*)

Dull aching pain in the abdomen, worse round the umbilicus. (*Dubs.*)

Colic-like pains in, and around the navel, every day. (*Dubs.*)

Dull aching pain in the right side of the abdomen, the whole afternoon, on a small spot. (*Neidhard.*)

Pain round the navel like colic, repeatedly, but always after the symptoms in the head. (*Neidhard.*)

145. Flatulent colic, like as if he had eaten unripe fruit, on waking up at night, below the navel, which is increased by movement after getting up; the pain diminishes during rest and returns periodically. (The night after taking it. *E. Smith.*)

In the morning after breakfast, on walking about, the same pain returns, gets better about 9 o'clock, and disappears entirely at 12 o'clock. (*E. Smith.*)

Sensation of soreness on touching, all around the navel. (*E. Smith.*)

Sensation of soreness in the abdomen. (*Neidhard.*)

Pain in the abdomen. *Christison.* (First felt six hours after swallowing half an ounce of oxalic acid, diluted in water.)

150. Sharp and constant pain in the left iliac region. (*Dubs.*)

For half an hour after retiring, a continued pain in the left hypochondrium. (*Neidhard.*)

A sticking pain in the left hypochondrium. (After three hours. *Williamson.*)

Pain between hypochondrium and navel, on the left side, like a development of flatulency. (In half an hour. (*Neidhard.*)

On sitting down after a walk, violent effort to discharge flatulency. (As from a small spot on the left iliac region.) Sensation as if the part would burst (*Neidhard.*)

Eructations and discharge of flatulency. 114.

155. Distressed feeling and great weakness in the whole abdomen, with flatulent colic. (*Dubs.*)

Great flatulency the whole day, with expulsion of wind downwards. Swelling of the abdomen with dull colic like pains *at intervals*, in and around the umbilicus, but worse in the right iliac region. Itching at the anus, with crawling sensation as if from worms, and which was relieved by rubbing the parts for several minutes. It returned several times during the night. (*Dubs.*)

Colic pain around the umbilicus, and in the right iliac region, coming on by paroxysms. (*Dubs.*)

Pain in the region of navel, with painful pressing down towards the anus and flatulency. (*Neidhard.*)

Pain in the region of the navel, with emission of flatulency in the night. (*Neidhard.*)

160. Difficult discharge of flatulency. (*Hering.*)

The whole evening rumbling in the bowels with pressing downwards. (*Neidhard.*)

Pain in the descending colon, followed by a free evacuation of mushy stool in the evening, one hour after taking it. (*Williamson.*)

A similar pain returned the second evening. (*Williamson.*)

6 o'clock, A. M., was suddenly seized with a distressing feeling in the whole abdomen, followed in several minutes by twisting in and around the umbilicus, with a discharge in a few minutes of a small quantity of hard fæces of a dark brown colour. In half an hour again violent pain and bearing down, followed by a loose evacuation, of a muddy-brown colour, accompained by colic pains in the navel. Below the navel he felt a bearing down, and griping pains in the anus. The latter were so severe, as to produce severe nervous pains through the head, with heat in this organ. After retiring to bed the same pains returned again in five minutes, followed by a copious evacuation of consistent dark muddy brown fæces. On going to bed the pains invariably returned, whilst sitting or reclining. Is better during motion. (Had to take merc. sol. 2*d*, to be relieved of the pain. *Dubs.*)

165. Violent symptoms of irritation in the alimentary canal. *Christison.* (From two drachms.)

Severe pain in the bowels, and frequent inclination to stool. *Christison.* (In a patient, who lived 13 hours after swallowing the poison.)

In the anus a dull slow stitch, often returning. (*Hering.*)

In the evening a slight pinching from flatulency near the anus. (*Hering.*)

On rising, a violent tenesmus in the upper part of the rectum, a prolonged, very painful urging from above downwards. (*Hering.*)

170. On sitting down to stool in the morning, pressing cutting pain from the right side of the rectum above, towards the anus. (*Hering.*)

Evacuation pappy, light-brown. (2d day. *Hering.*)

In the afternoon again, passage from the bowels, pappy, thick and short. During the passage violent stitches in the fleshy part of the left thumb, like little quick cuts of a knife. (*Hering.*) Comp. 224.

After the passage, a heavy rumbling in the right side of the abdomen, (cæcum,) and noise from flatulency. (2d day. *Hering.*)

Twice passage of the bowels during the day. (*Neidhard.*) Comp. 138.

175. Constant involuntary discharge of fluid fæces, occasionally mixed with blood. *Christison.*

Constipation. Christison, (in two persons who recovered.) Comp. 128.

During yawning, a pressing stitch above the right hip, which takes away his breath. (*Hering.*)

During hiccup a sticking pressure above the right hip. (*Hering.*) Comp. 116.

In the evening slight pain in the region of the right kidney. (*Neidhard.*)

URINE, GENITALS.—180. Disposition to pass water every two hours, and in large quantities. (2d day. *Dubs.*)

Inclination to pass water every hour, and in large quantities each time. Slight burning in passing the urine, which is clear, and of a straw colour. (3d day. *Dubs.*)

Profuse flow of light coloured urine frequently during the evening. (*Dubs.*)

Copious discharge of urine, at 5 o'clock in the morning. (*Williamson.*)

Urging to pass water, with copious discharge; the water is of a lighter colour than usual. (*Neidhard.*)

185. Desire to urinate; the urine is of a lighter colour. (2d day. *Hering.*)

Discharges less urine than usual. (1st day. *Hering.*)

Great increase of sexual desire during the night and morning, with voluptuous dreams every night, for three nights. (*Dubs.*) Comp. 37.

Excessive sexual desire. (5th day. *Dubs.*)

Excitement of the sexual function, repeatedly. (*Neidhard.*)

190. After walking out, pain in the testicles and

spermatic chord, more in the latter, and worse in the right side. (1st day. *Hering.*)

On lying down, erections, without any cause, and afterwards the pains in the testicles, mentioned above. (*Hering.*)

Sensation of contusion in both testicles. (*Neidhard.*)

During walking in the evening, a pretty severe pain and heaviness in both testicles, shooting along the spermatic chords; worse on the right side. (*Neidhard.*)

Jerking in the testicles and spermatic chord. (*Neidhard.*)

LARYNX and CHEST.—195. On walking in the open air tickling in the larynx, with a sensation of sticking, he coughs several times, the larynx feels swelled. (*Floto.*)

A natural secretion of mucus from the throat is diminished. (*Floto.*)

Expectoration of hard mucus in lumps, and watery running from the nose, with sneezing. (*Floto.*) Comp. 95.

Expectoration of thick yellow mucus from the throat. 110.

Hawking up of thick yellowish white phlegm with a black lump in the centre, of the size of a pea. (1st day. *Dubs.*)

* The chronic sore throat, to which he is subject, is much better. 109.

During speaking, a sensation of mucus in the larynx, hoarseness; he has to expectorate more than usual. (*Hering.*)

Augments, the 1st hour, the secretion of mucus from the throat. 111.

200. Slight cough, from tickling in the larynx and trachea; also sensation of soreness in the larynx. (*Neidhard.*)

Difficulty of breathing, with constrictive pain in the larynx, and wheezing; oppression of the whole chest towards the right side. (*Floto.*)

Sharp shooting pain in the left lung and heart, extending down to the epigastrium, lasting for some seconds. (From 5 grs. 1-10*th*. 4th day. *Dubs.*)

In the afternoon, stitches several times in the left lung. (5th day. *Dubs.*)

Stitches in the left breast, more during walking. (*Floto.*)

205. Sharp, lancinating pain in the left lung, coming on so suddenly, that it deprived him of breath for several seconds, and then gradually subsided. (6th day. *Dubs.*)

In the forenoon, during repose, and also afterwards, during walking, a pain in the heart, extending from behind and below towards the anterior part. The pain in the heart is very violent, like electric flashes coming from within. (*Hering.*)

Immediately after lying down in bed at night, palpitation of the heart, for half an hour, three nights consecutively. (*Neidhard.*)

LOINS and BACK.—After rising from the recumbent position, a pain in the region of the loins towards the right, between the last rib and hip. (*Hering.*)

Weakness in the loins and hips, extending down to the lower extremities. (From 5 grs. 1-10*th*. *Dubs.*)

210. Pain, shooting down from the loins to the limbs, the patient seeking constant relief in a change of posture. *Christison.* (In a patient, who died in thirteen hours.)

The pain in the sacrum, habitual to him in the morning, is gone; instead of it a bruised sensation in the back from the loins to the shoulders. (2d day. *Hering.*)

Acute pain in the back, gradually extending down to the thighs, occasioning ere long great torture, and continuing almost to the moment of death. *Christison.* (The first symptom in a patient who had swallowed half an ounce of ox. ac. He died in thirteen hours.)

Numbness and weakness in the back and limbs. Christison.

Sense of numbness and tingling or pricking in the

back and thighs. *Christison.* (From two scruples, in 24 hours.)

215. Sensation of numbness in sacrum. (*Neidhard.*)

Creeping of cold, particularly from the lower part of the spine upwards. 37.

ARMS and LEGS.—Sharp shooting pain in the right shoulder-joint, coming on suddenly, and lasting about 15 minutes. (One hour after 3 grs. 1-10*th.* *Dubs.*)

After lying down in bed, a twitch in the left deltoid muscle, and in a few minutes one in the right. (*Kitchen.*)

During the forenoon increased sprain-like pain in the right wrist, which he has had for some time. (1st day. *Hering.*)

The pain in the right wrist worse; it jars and cracks. (2d day. *Hering.*)

220. *The right wrist painful, as if it were strained or dislocated.* On taking hold of any thing, he has to let it fall again. (3d day. *Hering.*)

During writing, a violent jerking pain in the ulnar region, near the right metacarpus. (1st day. *Hering.*)

Sensation of slight numbness in the left arm. (*Hering.*)

Sensation as if the hands were dead. *Christison.*

Tensive pain in the fleshy part of the left thumb, with heat, numbness, and a sensation of swelling, lasting about half an hour. (After 30 minutes. *Kitchen.*)

Lividity of the nails and fingers. Comp. 50.

225. Sticking pain in the right hip-joint. (*Williamson.*)

Aching pain in the right ankle-joint, with a feeling of swelling, of this part and the whole right foot. (From 5 grs. 1-10*th.* *Dubs.*)

Sharp shooting pain on the instep of the right foot, lasting for half an hour, at intervals. (*Dubs.*)

The same pain the next day, lasting five minutes. (*Dubs.*)

Sharp pain in the right ankle-joint, several days after the first pain. (*Dubs.*)

230. *A very violent contracting pain in the external tendon of the left knee.* (1st day. *Hering.*)

Jerking, sliding pain in the hollow of the left knee. (*Hering.*)

Uneasiness in limbs and feet, which he is hardly able to keep quiet for a few minutes at a time. (*Dubs.*)

Slight lameness and stiffness in the lower extremities. (*Neidhard.*)

Lividity, coldness, and almost complete loss of the power of motion in the legs, which symptoms were not entirely removed for fifteen days. *Christison.* (From two drachms.)

ELATERIUM.

BY CALEB B. MATTHEWS, M. D.

Momordica elaterium—Wild or Squirting Cucumber—Its Inspissated Juice—The Extract of the Fruit.

Synon. Concombre sauvage, (Fr.)—Eselsgurken, (Germ.)

Nat. Ord. Cucurbitaceæ.

Sex. Syst. Monoecia, Syngenesia.

GEN. CHAR.—*Flowers* monoecious white or yellow, with a filiform peduncle having one bract. MALES: *calyx* five-cleft, with a very short tube. *Corol.* five-parted. *Stam.* triadelphous; *anthers* connate. FEMALES: *filaments* three or five, triadelphous, sterile. *Style* three-cleft. *Ovar.* bilocular. *Fruit* muricate, opening with elasticity when ripe. *Seeds* compressed, reticulated when ripe.

SP. CHAR.—Hisped-rough, glaucous. *Stem* short, without tendrils. *Flowers* axillary. *Leaves* cordate, somewhat lobed, crenate dentate, very rugose on long petioles. *Fruit* ovate, obtuse, hispid-rough, with long peduncles. *Seeds* chesnut-brown. *Root* annual.

The experiments from which the following symptoms were obtained, were made with the pellets moistened with the second dilution, prepared from the extract of elaterium, first by trituration with sac. lactis, and then by dilution in alcohol in the proportions to form the second dilution. Twenty or thirty pellets were given and evinced the same symptoms in several individuals on whom it was tried, very soon after its administration.

The elaterium of the shops is liable to one inconvenience; it is found sometimes to be very inferior, if not entirely inert; and others, in making the dilutions, may, from that circumstance, fail to produce the desired results.

"The judicious experiments of Dr. Clutterbuck prove that the active principle of the Momordica elaterium resides more particularly in the juice, which is lodged in the centre of the fruit, (around the seeds) and which spontaneously subsides from it."* Dr. Clutterbuck obtained only six grains of *genuine* elaterium from forty wild cucumbers, and of this an *eighth* part of *a grain* seldom failed to purge violently, "yet, strange as it may appear, not more than *one grain in ten* of elaterium, as it occurs in commerce, possesses any active properties; and that this decimal part is a vegetable proximate principle, not hitherto noticed,"† called by Paris *Elatin.*

The early history of elaterium, which appears from Dioscorides and others to have been employed with much confidence and success, by the ancients, is involved in great confusion; some authors speaking of different preparations by that name. Hippocrates uses the term elaterium to mean *any* violent purgative.

The elaterium of Dioscorides is presumed to be the article at present in use. He states its dose to be from gr. ij. to ℈j.; Ætius, Paulus, and Actuarius recommend ʒss.; Mesue, ℈ss. to ℈j.; Bontius, ℈j. to ʒss.; while Massarius gives doses of grs. vj.; Herman from grs. v. to grs. vij.; Quincy, grs. v.; Boerhaave, grs. iv.; and the physicians of the present times give from grs. ss., to grs. ij. These discrepancies, while they show the uncertainty of the article, are to be explained, as shown by Clutterbuck's experiments, on the principle of different degrees of admixture of inert matter in the specimens used by different practitioners. I have found it act on the bowels, producing several discharges, in doses of the 20th of a grain, triturated with refined loaf sugar.

* Paris' Pharmacologia, page 258. † Ibid. page 270.

The elaterium of commerce comes to us in small thin cakes, having the impression of the muslin on which it was placed to dry. It is of a greenish colour, and bitter somewhat acrid taste. The purest is light, pulverulent, and inflammable.

Paris, in his Pharmacologia, (page 272,) states that there is a *bitter* principle in the elaterium very distinct from the extractive matter, having no purgative property whatever; but when taken only produces an increased appetite—yet when combined with the elatin, the latter is much accelerated in its action by the presence of the former.

The dose of good elaterium used by physicians of the old school, as a hydragogue for which it has principally been heretofore employed, in the cure of dropsy in its various forms, especially hydrothorax, is from half to two grains.

It differs from most other powerful cathartics, in exciting the pulse and producing *febrile* action. It has occasionally produced great prostration, and even death from its imprudent use, and was in consequence banished from practice, until its use was revived by Dr. Ferriar, of Manchester, with great success in the cure of hydrothorax.

From the foregoing brief account of elaterium, it will be perceived that though it has been used at intervals for twenty centuries, yet little has been known of its properties, except that of a powerful and dangerous purgative; and this fact establishes the superior advantages to be derived from the homœopathic method of investigating the character of remedies.

Even from the following brief detail of symptoms, the intelligent physician can perceive at once various forms of disease to which this remedy is applicable, and can employ it both with safety and certainty. It appears to have analogous action to nux vomica and veratrum, especially the latter. Always regarding the fundamental law of homœopathia, the diseases to which elaterium appears to be adapted are,—bilious fevers, diarrhœas, especially after cholera; cholera morbus;

intermittents; rheumatism; arthritis; cephalalgia, especially connected with flatulence; indigestion, and hepatic diseases; and I have accordingly found it so in practice, as the cases detailed in the succeeding appendix to this article will confirm.

Incessant gaping, lasting for nearly an hour.

Sharp, fugitive, or dull aching pains now here, now there.

Pains mostly affecting the left side, but also the right.

Chilliness with continued gaping, as if an attack of intermittent fever was approaching.

5. Depression of spirits.

Fear of some approaching disaster.

Dull pain in the region of causality.

Dull pains in the region of combativeness, right and left sides.

Pains in the temples.

10. Sticking as of a splinter, in the inner canthus of the left eye.

Sticking pain near the rim of the cartilage of the left ear.

Bitter taste in the mouth.

A feeling as if the choana and upper part of the œsophagus was enlarged.

Sharp pains at the lower part of the sternum, passing through to the spine or lower angle of the right shoulder blade.

15. Rumbling of flatus, in the course of the cœcum and colon.

Dull pains in the bowels.

Watery discharges from the bowels of a frothy character.

Discharges of dark masses of bilious mucus.

Dull olive green discharges.

20. Costiveness.

Dull pain in the epigastrium.

Feeling of stricture or oppression at the epigastrium.

Cutting pains in the bowels, like the griping of medicine.

Dull pain in the right hypochondrium.

25. Constant nausea and disposition to vomit.

Eructations of flatus.

Pain of a dull aching, pressing kind over the crest of the right ilium, round to the back, extending deep into the pelvis.

Bleeding of hæmorrhoidal tumours.

Discharge of flatus, per anum.

30. Increased flow of limpid urine.

Pains under the right shoulder blade.

Pains in the left sterno-cleido-mastoideus muscle, near its insertion into the sternum.

Fugitive sticking pains in the lumbar region, more on the right side.

Sharp shooting pains in the left axilla, near the insertion of the pectoralis major muscle.

35. Pains extending from the shoulder to the ends of the fingers, and shooting back, up to the elbow.

Sharp sticking pains in the muscular parts of the thumb.

Sharp sticking pains in the fingers of the left hand, out to their extremities.

Dull pains in the right shoulder, forearm and hand, extending to the fingers.

Shooting and also dull aching pains in the left thigh, in the course of the sciatic nerve, extending down to the instep, and out to the extremities of the toes.

40. Pain in the right knee, extending into the instep and toes.

Pain in the great toe of an arthritic nature.

APPENDIX.

Febris biliosa. ——, captain of a canal boat, who, in August, had passed through the Pennsylvania canals, was soon after attacked with fever, followed by cutting pains in the bowels, watery discharges, accompanied by nausea and vomiting, was cured by two doses of the elaterium. Dose 10 pellets of the 2*d dilution.*

Febris biliosa. ——, a hand, on board the same canal boat, as the above case. Burning fever, cutting pains in the bowels, vomiting and purging of watery dejections. The same dose of elaterium was given, and the purging occurred but once after its use, and in the afternoon he had recovered so far as to leave the boat, and the next day was able to assist in his ordinary duties.

Diarrhœa. Wm. Myers, was labouring under ascites and anasarca, during which he was attacked with watery diarrhœa, with cutting pains in the bowels; two doses of elaterium, ten pellets of the 2*d*, arrested the diarrhœa, and allayed the pain. Some weeks after, the symptoms again recurred, and the same remedy afforded similar relief.

Diarrhœa. Mr. ——, had been partially relieved of cholera morbus, with cutting pains, vomiting and purging of watery fluids, by veratrum. The diarrhœa continued; elaterium, ten pellets of the 2*d* dilution, was given and repeated several times at intervals of two hours; a speedy cure was the result.

Dysenteria biliosa. A child of Mr. Pleis, aged about 5 years, soon after having passed safely through the measles, from exposure to damp weather was attacked with dysentery, presenting the following symptoms: Discharges very frequent, with much pain in the abdomen, and constant urging to stool. The dejections partly composed of masses of dark green mucus, with portions of whitish mucus tinged with blood. Several apparently indicated remedies were given, with but partial, if any relief. Elaterium, in the 2*d* dilution, about twenty pellets to a wine-glassfull of water, and a teaspoonful given every two hours, effected an entire cure.

Cholera morbus. Thomas Myers was attacked with watery diarrhœa, which in a few hours terminated in violent cholera morbus. It was apparently produced by standing on the damp ground after great bodily exertion.

The symptoms were violent cutting pains in the bowels, recurring at intervals of ten or fifteen minutes; frequent stools of a watery nature, with vomiting; the disease had lasted all night; and the next morning until 11 o'clock, when I saw him; he had used cayenne pepper and whiskey externally, and several drops of oil of camphor internally without relief. Veratrum in the 3*d* dilution, ten pellets given on the tongue, failed. In half an hour after taking the elaterium in the same manner, ten pellets of the 2*d*, he was relieved and fell asleep; vomiting ceased. The remedy was repeated several times on account of the diarrhœa. After three or four stools without pain, he was entirely cured by the middle of the afternoon, and went to his ordinary avocations next morning.

Cholera morbus. Miss —— aged about 25 years, was attacked with cholera morbus, cutting pains in the abdomen, fluid stools, nausea and vomiting, accompained with a feeling of oppression, stricture and pain in the epigastrium, and difficult breathing; a single dose of the elaterium in the 2*d* relieved her entirely. She had been previously subject to the oppression at the epigastrium, which appeared to arise from indigestion. She has been always relieved by the elaterium, a few pellets of the 2*d dilution*, being given.

Febris intermittens. Mr. ——, aged about 56 years, had been labouring under quartan ague for six weeks, the paroxysms occurring at about 12 o'clock, M.; when an attack resembling cholera morbus supervened, and I was called to visit him. He laboured under a severe and copious discharge of frothy fluid matter, frequently dejected from the bowels, with cutting pains at intervals, and vomiting; veratrum 3*d* was given with partial relief to the violent symptoms. Elaterium 2*d*, at intervals of two or three hours, effected an entire cure of the symptoms of cholera, in a few hours, and when the proper period arrived for the recurrence of his ague, he found he was also cured of that, and has remained well.

Febris intermittens. Mrs. ——, aged 35 years, had

laboured under a very obstinate tertian ague for about five years, which she had contracted while residing in Virginia. It was suppressed at intervals by sulph. quinine, in large doses, but always recurred at longer or shorter periods. When the chills were suppressed she was generally attacked with urticaria, over the whole surface, and she frequently was afflicted with a disordered state of mind, characterized by an irresistible propensity to wander from home, even in the night, and range in the woods, &c. The symptoms, when I was called to treat her, were as follows: chill every third day, twice in the day, continuing two hours; pains in the head; under the shoulder blades; in the left side; in the calves of the legs and small of the back; yawning and gaping with a sound resembling the neighing of a horse; running at the nose; cramps in the legs and soles of the feet. The chill was followed by high fever, which ended in copious perspiration.

The elaterium cured the ague perfectly after other of the apparently adapted remedies had failed. Dose ten pellets of the 2*d*, every three hours, repeated for some days, during which there were several recurring paroxysms.

Urticaria. After the ague had subsided in the above case, urticaria appeared, with tendency of mind above stated, a continuance of the elaterium for a few days entirely and permanently removed this latter affection and she has had no recurrence.

About twenty minutes after taking the medicine it produced a great heat under the shoulder blades, and free spitting of large lumps of yellow matter, apparently from the stomach. This lady found that when she took large doses of the elaterium, about fifty pellets of the 2*d*, or one-third of a teaspoonful, it acted on the bowels, overcame costiveness and aggravated the gaping.

My friend, Dr. Jeanes, has used the elaterium at my suggestion, and has kindly furnished me with the following cases of intermittent fever.

"*Febris intermittens tertiana.* J. Houston, aged 28

years, had first quotidian ague, which was repeatedly suppressed for a few days by Rowand's Tonic Mixture, until the medicine appeared no longer to exert any control over the disease, which at the time of his calling upon me was of the tertain type.

The paroxysms were preceded by much gaping, and were attended by much thirst, with pain in the abdomen, and great pain in the extremities, darting down into the fingers and toes. Three powders, each containing a drop of the 3*d dilution*, were given, to be taken before the next paroxysm, at intervals of twelve hours. The first paroxysm after the medicine, was less severe than those before, and the next, which was the last, was very slight. Since that time, now more than three months, he has remained free from the disease.

Febris intermittens quotidiana. T. M. C., aged 30 years. Intermittent fever contracted eighteen months since in Virginia, and suppressed every one, two or three weeks, by the use or abuse of quinine.

Paroxysms preceded by headache, soreness of the limbs; pains in the bowels; continued gaping and stretching. In the chill, slightly increased pain in the head and limbs. In the fever, violent tearing pains throughout the head, but most in the region of benevolence; increased pain in the bowels and extremities; the pains shoot to the very tips of the fingers and toes, and then shoot back into the body; the thirst intense. In the sweat, all the symptoms gradually subside. Access at one o'clock, P. M.

A dose of elaterium, eight pellets of the 2*d dilution*, in the evening after the cessation of the sweat, and another of the same in the morning, was followed by a severe paroxysm, but presenting considerable variation from those which preceded the employment of the medicine. The next paroxysm was very light, and the third and last was barely perceptible. No other doses than the two above mentioned were given."

Icterus neonatorum.—The author of this article was called to see the child of Mrs. Wallace, about the third day after its birth. It was afflicted with jaundice; the skin over the whole body of an orange yellow; the whites of the eyes deeply tinged; the urine stained the diaper, and the stools were bilious. One pellet of the 2d *dilution*, three times a day, was given for three or four days, when a rapid and permanent cure resulted.

Colica flatulenta. Mr. George K——, aged 84 years, while labouring under an attack of obstinate diarrhœa, for which he was treated homœopathically and was relieved by other remedies, suffered from a flatulent colic which supervened, and was attended with borborigmus, and severe pain in the lower part of the abdomen. He was speedily relieved by a few pellets of the 2*d dilution* dissolved in a wineglass of water, and a teaspoonful given every hour.

Colica flatulenta. A child of Mrs. Evans, aged five years, attacked with cramp-like pains in the abdomen and chest, accompanied with costiveness, was cured by taking a few doses of the pellets of the 2*d dilution*, of elaterium. Warm watery injections were, however, used in aid of the remedy.

Rheumatismus sciatica. A. ——, aged about 25 years, was attacked with this disease, characterized by tearing and gnawing pains in the hips and thighs, deeply seated. She was relieved completely in two days, by the elaterium. The dose was five pellets of the 2*d dilution*, three times a day.

Biliary calculi. Miss B. aged about 60, applied to me to relieve a pain in the right hypochondrium, and dull pain in the epigastrium. She used the 2*d dilution*, in the form of pellets three times a day. After some days she discharged from the bowels a considerable quantity of a gravelly substance, which was readily discernable after washing the fæces with water; this continued for several days, with great relief to the patient and a removal of the pains preceding the occurrence.

Indigestion.—Jas. Le Count, aged about 70 years, was attacked with bitter taste in the mouth, dull pain in the epigastrium; pains in the head, especially in the region of combativeness on both sides, with dull pains in the temples; nausea. He was completely cured by a single dose of elaterium, 2*d dilution*, ten pellets.

Neuralgia. Mrs. T——, of Baltimore, was attacked with paralysis of the left side, accompanied with acute neuralgic pains in the right side, extreme pain in the right temple, shoulder, arm and over the crest of the right os ilium and down the thighs; with bitter taste in the mouth; suppression of urine; rheumatic pain and swelling of the right knee of a sub-acute nature. During her treatment for this complaint, purging and vomiting occurred, which was relieved by veratrum, but the neuralgic pains and suppression of urine were decidedly relieved by the elaterium, 2*d dilution*, fifteen pellets in a wineglass of water, and a teaspoonful given every two hours.

Many other cases of the various diseases above stated might be given, but it was deemed unnecessary to swell this article by repetitions of similar details. Enough it is hoped has been presented to show that the elaterium is a remedy of great value, and deserving of a more elaborate investigation.

EUPATORIUM PERFOLIATUM.

BY W. WILLIAMSON, M. D.

Synon. Eupatorium connatum; Eupatorium virginianum; Eupatorium foliis connatis tomentosis.

Vulgo. Bone-set; Thorough-wort; Thorough stem; Cross-wort; Thorough-wax; Vegetable Antimony; Indian sage; Ague-weed; Joe-pye.

German. Durchwachsener Wasserdost.

Nat. Syst. Juss. Corymbiferæ.

Nat. Ord. Lin. Compositæ discoideæ.

Art. Syst. Lin.—CLASS. Syngenesia.

ORDER. Polygamia aequalis.

GEN. CHAR.—*Calyx* oblong, imbricate or rarely simple; scales linear-lanceolate, erect, unequal, unarmed.

Corol. Compound, uniform, discoid; florets all uniform, perfect, fertile, monopetalous, funnel-shaped, with a regular five-cleft spreading border.

Stam. Filaments five, capillary very short; anthers united into a cylindrical tube.

Pist. Germ minute; style thread-shaped, very long, much exsert, cloven half way down, slender, bluntish, straight.

Peric. None, except the permanent calyx.

Seeds. Solitary, oblong, five-striate, smooth and glandular; down long, rough or feathery.

Recep. Naked.

SPEC. CHAR.—Leaves connate-perfoliate, broadest at the base, oblong-serrate, acuminate, rugose, rough, narrow above, tomentose beneath, decussate; the two or three upper pairs of leaves are sessile; under surface paler than the upper; stem villous, erect, round, from two to four feet high, and divided towards the top into decussating branches, of a greyish-green colour, but often purplish towards the base. Flowers terminal, white, in fastigiate corymbs on short hairy peduncles; florets twelve or fourteen in number. Anthers deep blue or black. Seeds black, pappus pilose. The root is perennial, and grows nearly horizontal. Blooms from the latter end of July to the beginning of November, and grows throughout North America, in meadows and other low grounds, along the course of small streams, &c.; generally in small patches, but occasionally covering an acre or more of ground.

The genus is called Eupatorium, in honour of Mithridates, surnamed Eupator, who is said to have discovered the original plant, and used it as an antidote against poisons.

There are about seventy species of Eupatorium enumerated by Botanists, thirty-three of which number are indigenous to North America.

The leaves and the flowers are the parts of the plant generally used for medicinal purposes and mostly in the form of tincture, made with some spirituous menstruum, by which its active properties appear to be fully extracted. Alleopathists frequently use it in decoction, cold infusion, or in powder.

It emits a faint odour, and possesses an exceedingly bitter and somewhat peculiar taste.

Chemically, Eupatorium perfoliatum contains a free acid, tannin, a bitter extractive matter, a gummy matter, resin, nitrogen, lime probably in the state of acetate, gallic acid, a resiniform matter soluble in water and alcohol containing a bitter principle. It yields a salifiable base, which forms, with sulphuric acid, crystals of a prismatic shape, and tasteless, called Eupatoria.

This, like many other indigenous plants, has been extolled for a time for its medicinal virtues, and then in its turn passed by with indifference, or perhaps rejected on account of the extravagant encomiums bestowed upon it by its advocates. Notwithstanding the vacillating course of the profession generally in relation to its merits, there ever have been highly respectable practitioners who have appreciated its real worth, and considered it one of the most useful articles of the Materia Medica.

The various classifications of the eupatorium by different writers, manifest its diversified action. We find it associated with tonics, stimulants, diaphoretics, emetics, cathartics, diuretics, astringents, deobstruents, &c. &c.; and accordingly we hear of its effective agency in the cure of intermittent and remittent fevers, yellow fever, spotted fever, typhus fever, typhoid pneumonia, rheumatism, gout, catarrhs, influenza, dropsy, dyspepsia, cutaneous diseases, &c.

It is said to have been very successful in the treatment of a peculiar herpetic disease, affecting the anus and adjacent parts, as the scrotum and thighs, and also sometimes extending its ravages to the rectum; endemic along James River, in Virginia, and from that circumstance called the James River ring-worm.

A wine-glassfull of the expressed juice of the plant taken every hour, and the bruised leaves applied to the part, is celebrated as a cure for the bite of the rattle snake.

Nearly half a century ago there prevailed throughout the United States, but particularly in the state of Pennsylvania, a peculiar epidemic, which, from the constancy of the attending symptom of pain in the bones, was called *break bone fever*. The Eupatorium perfoliatum, although a diaphoretic, so signally relieved the disease, notwithstanding *copious perspiration* was a frequent attendant, that it was familiarly called *bone-set;* a common name, by which it is still extensively known.

This herb is one of the remedies, and perhaps the principal one employed by the aborigines of this country, in the treatment of intermittent fevers, and hence another of the common names by which it is known among us—"ague-weed,"—which corresponds to the Indian name.

In miasmatic districts, along rivers, at fisheries, on

marshes and their several neighbourhoods, where intermittent and remittent fevers have prevailed epidemically, the eupatorium has been a favourite remedy with the most successful practitioners, as well as a deservedly popular one in the hands of the people ; very often superceding the necessity of calling in medical aid, especially where such aid could not readily be obtained.

In all cases of low typhoid disease, attended with hot, dry skin, it is reputed to be an estimable medicine.

It was used with great success in an epidemic of influenza, and lake fever, which prevailed a few years ago in the neighbourhood of Lake Ontario.

In 1812 it was substituted for peruvian bark in the treatment of intermittent fevers in the New York Almshouse, and with uniform success.

When physicians of the old school wish to have the tonic (?) effect of eupatorium, they give the powdered leaves and flowers in substance, or if they wish to produce diaphoresis, they give it in decoction, and increase the dose in order to procure emesis.

It is remarkable, that the Eupatorium perfoliatum, when given in large doses, produces very *copious diaphoresis*, and yet one of the indications for its use in the treatment of intermittent fevers, homœopathically, appears to be *inconsiderable perspiration.*

Those symptoms in the following enumeration not accredited to any authority, are to be understood as belonging to the writer of this monograph.

Compare with: Arn., Cham., Merc., Natr. mur., Rhus tox., Tar. em. It alternates well with Natr. mur., in intermittent fevers.

The cases in which this medicine promises the greatest usefulness appear to be :

Headache, arising from disordered stomach.

Nervous headache—hemicrania.

Fevers, attended with gastric derangement.

Intermittent fever, especially when the paroxysm occurs in the morning.

Remittent fever, of miasmatic origin or typhoid character.

Bilious fever.

Rheumatic affections, accompanied by perspiration, and soreness of the bones.

Gouty affections.

Cachectic condition of the system from long continued or frequent attacks of bilious and intermittent fevers.

Indigestion of old people.

Dyspepsia.

Loss of appetite.

General debility.

Bronchitis.

Tardy developement of eruptive diseases, and especially measles.

Nocturnal cough, particularly after the eruptive stage of measles.

Dropsical affections.

Influenza, with weakness of the pulse and great prostration of the system.

Influenza of old people and inebriates.

HEAD.—Headache with the sensation of soreness internally; better in the house; aggravated when first going into the open air; relieved by conversation.

Pain extending from the forehead to the occiput; greatest in the left side.

* Throbbing headache. (*Neidhard.*)

* Headache and sick stomach, every other morning when first getting awake, which continues all day, with loss of appetite during the headache, but good appetite on the intervening day.

5. Beating pain in the nape and occiput; better after rising.

* Pain in the occiput after lying, with the sensation of

a great weight in the part, requiring the assistance of the hands to lift it.

Darting pains through the temples, with the sensation of blood rushing *across* the head.

* Distress on the top and in the back part of the head.

* Shooting pains from the left to the right side of the head.

10. * Painful soreness in the right parietal protuberance.

Heat on the top of the head, with pain, which is relieved by pressure.

* Thumping in the side of the head, above the right ear.

* Soreness and beating in the back part of the head.

EYES.—Soreness of the eye-balls.

15. * Intolerance of light.

Redness of margins of the lids, with glutinous secretion from the meibomian glands.

Increased lacrymation.

* Pain and soreness in the left eye-ball.

NOSE.—* Flowing coryza.

20. * Sneezing.

FACE.—* Sickly, sallow countenance.

Flushed face.

Redness of the cheeks, with dry skin.

MOUTH.—Paleness of the mucous membrane of the mouth.

25. * Tongue coated, yellow. (*Neidhard.*)

Tongue covered with white fur.

* Sores in the corners of the mouth.

THROAT.—Dryness of the throat.

* Soreness of fauces, with catarrh.

APPETITE.—30. Insipid taste in the mouth.

* Tastelessness of food. (*Neidhard.*)

* Want of appetite. (*Neidhard.*)

Loss of appetite.

Distaste for food.

35. Nocturnal thirst for something cold.

Thirst for cold water.

Desire for ice cream.

STOMACH.—Belching of tasteless wind, with a feeling of obstruction at the pit of the stomach.

Sensation of something in the stomach that ought to come up, without the ability to raise it.

40. General shuddering, proceeding from the stomach.

Sensation of fulness in the stomach.

Beating in the epigastrium in the night.

Heat in the stomach.

Nausea and vomiting of food.

45. * *Vomiting immediately after drinking.*

Vomiting preceded by thirst.

* *Vomiting of bile, with trembling, attended by pain in the epigastrium, with nausea and extreme prostration,* almost syncope.

Distressing disposition to vomit.

Nausea and vomiting with free perspiration, and copious expectoration.

50. Qualmishness from odours; the smell of food cooking, &c.

ABDOMEN.—* Soreness around the waist.

Tight clothing is oppressive.

Soreness and fulness in the region of the liver.

Tightness in the left hypochondrium.

BOWELS.—55. * Constipation.

* Costiveness attending catarrh.

Purging stools, with smarting and heat in the anus.

Tenesmus, with a small discharge of loose stool.

Morning diarrhœa.

60. Four or five watery stools in the day.

URINE.—Urine scanty, and high coloured.

Copious evacuation of limpid urine.

* Dark brown scanty urine, depositing a whitish clay like sediment; voided but once in twenty-four hours.

Dark coloured clear urine.

65. * Itching of the mons veneris.

LARYNX.—* Hoarseness, with roughness in the voice.

Hacking cough in the evening.

Cough, with soreness and heat in the bronchia.

Cough, aggravated in the evening.

70. * Hectic cough from suppressed intermittent fever.

* Nocturnal loose cough.

* Hoarse rough cough, with scraping in the bronchia.

* Violent cough, with soreness in the chest.

* Cough, with flushed face and tearful eyes—the patient supports his chest with the hands.

75. * Cough preceding measles.

* Cough following measles.

* Disposition to cough, with dyspnœa.

CHEST.—* Dyspnœa very great, obliging the patient to lie with his head and shoulders very high.

* Difficulty of breathing, attended with perspiration, and anxious countenance; with sleepiness.

80. * Painful irritation of the pulmonary organs, with heat in the chest.

Aching pain under the left breast.

Inability to lie on the left side.

Soreness in the chest, from taking a full inspiration.

* Deep-seated pain in the left side and in the right shoulder.

85. Grating sensation in the chest, at every deep inspiration.

TRUNK.—Weakness in the small of the back.

Deep-seated pain in the loins, with soreness from motion.

Pain in the back, as from a bruise.

Beating pain in the nape.

* Pain in the back and lower extremities.

UPPER EXTREMITIES.—90. Soreness and aching in the arms and forearms.

Stiffness of the arms.

Painful soreness in both wrists, as if broken or dislocated.

Stiffness of the fingers, with obtuseness of the sense of touch.

* Heat in the palms of the hands, sometimes with moisture.

LOWER EXTREMITIES.—95. * Pain in a spot not larger than a pea, over the left hip, with soreness.

Pain, with extreme sensitiveness in the left glutei muscles, passing round in front of the trochanter major.

* Burning in the skin, on the inner side of the thighs of a female.

* Flagging of the muscles of the left thigh, as if they were falling off the bone.

* Gouty inflammation of the left knee and the right elbow. The pains are worse from 10 o'clock, A. M., until 4 o'clock, P. M.

100. Pain and soreness of the upper part of the left foot, with increased sensibility of the left big toe.

The pain in the foot is increased by standing upon it.

Stiffness, and general soreness of the lower extremities, when rising to walk.

Calves of the legs feel as if they had been beaten.

* Soreness and swelling of both feet when standing on them, in a gouty subject.

105. Pain in the first joint of the left great toe which suddenly moves to the corresponding joint of the right one.

Pricking in the soles of the feet.

Aching pain in the right hip, while sitting.

* Lameness in the right hip and lower extremity, when walking.

Soreness and aching of the lower limbs.

110. * Throbbing in the right foot.

* Rheumatic pain on the inside of the left knee.

* Dropsical swelling of both feet and ankles.

Heat in the soles of the feet in the morning.

FEVER.—Intermittent fever, quotidian, tertian and quartan.

115. The paroxysm generally commences in the morning. *Thirst several hours before the chill, which continues during the chill and heat.*

Chilliness through the night, and in the morning, with nausea, from the least motion.

Aching pain and soreness, as if from having been beaten in the calves of the legs, small of the back and in the arms, above and below the elbows.

* Flushed face and dry hot skin, during the fever.

* Chill at 7 o'clock in the morning, preceded by thirst, and attended with moisture of the hands.

120. * *Vomiting at the conclusion of the chill.*

* Fever, accompanied with sleep and moaning, and followed by slight perspiration.

* The patient continues lying after the fever goes off.

* Nausea and sickness of the stomach, at the commencement of the heat, with violent throbbing headache, (*Neidhard.*)

* *Chill in the morning*, heat during the rest of the day, and *slight perspiration* in the evening. (*Neidhard.*)

125. * Intermittent fever with a heavy chill, early in the morning of one day, and a light chill about noon the next day, and so on successively.

* Headache and trembling during the heat.

* Chill preceded by pain above the right ilium, with thirst and a disposition to yawn.

* *Pain in the bones early in the morning before the paroxysm.*

* The chill is induced or hastened by taking a drink of water.

130. * Headache, back ache and thirst during the chill.

* *Nausea as the chill goes off.*

* Increased headache, but diminished thirst, during the heat.

Aching in the bones of the extremities, with soreness of the flesh.

* Coldness with a great deal of trembling, attended with nausea.

135. *Chilliness, with excessive trembling and nausea.*

* Internal trembling, with external heat.

Chilliness in the morning, heat throughout the rest of the day, but no perspiration.

* Coldness and stinging or pricking, as from pins, in both feet at the commencement of the chill.

* Aching in the bones of the extremities, in the latter part of the chill, and in the beginning of the heat.

140. The patient feels worse in the morning of one day, and in the afternoon of the next.

Nocturnal sweat with chilliness, from motion or removal of the covering.

* The thirst frequently commences in the *night previous* to the chill, in tertian ague.

* Chill begins at 9 o'clock in the morning.

* Stiffness of the fingers during the chill.

145. Soreness in the bones.

* Aching pain with moaning throughout the cold stage.

* *A greater amount of shivering during the chill, than is warranted by the degree of coldness.*

Retching and vomiting of bile.

Vomiting after every draught.

150. * *Vomiting at the conclusion of the chill.*

* Distressing pain in the scrobiculus cordis, throughout the chill and heat.

* *Throbbing headache during the chill and heat.*

* Violent pain in the head and back, before the chill.

* *Inconsiderable perspiration* or *none at all*, after the hot stage.

155. * Fever in the forenoon, preceded by thirst early in the morning, but no chill; attended by fatigueing cough, and not followed by perspiration.

* Loose cough in the intermission.

* Cough in the night previous to the paroxysm.

* Great weakness and prostration during the fever, with faintness from motion.

* The patient cannot raise his head from the pillow, while the fever lasts.

160. Trembling in the back during fever.

* The heat goes off by moderate perspiration, during sleep in the evening.

* Thirst throughout the night before the paroxysm, in tertian ague. *Thirst several hours before the chill.*

* The thirst continues during the chill and heat, with vomiting after each draught of water.

165. * Vomiting of bile at the close of the hot stage.

* Inconsiderable perspiration after the fever.

* Coldness during nocturnal perspiration.

Chilliness from motion.

Pungent heat attending the perspiration at night.

170. Alternate chilliness and flashes of heat.

* Fever, with despondency of mind, morbid sensitiveness of the skin, and sleeplessness.

APPENDIX.

I have observed the most decided effects from the Eupatorium perfoliatum, in the treatment of certain cases of intermittent fever; in two of which the following symptoms were present: violent thirst before the chill, and slight during it; nausea and sickness of the stomach, (in one case vomiting) at the commencement of the heat, with violent throbbing headache; tastelessness of food; want of appetite; tongue coated yellow; the chills set in in the morning, and lasted for one or two hours; heat during the rest of the day, and slight perspiration in the evening; type tertian. In one case the sulph. of quinine had been administered, without preventing the recurrence of the paroxysms.

I gave in the apyrexia gtt. 3 of the tinct. eup. p., in water, every hour, which produced no aggravation, a slight headache excepted, and prevented the return of the next attack permanently. (*Neidhard.*)

Case 1. I was called to Mrs. S——, who lived in a miasmatic district, on the 19th of November, 1841. Irregular quotidian. The chill generally began at nine o'clock, in the morning, and lasted four hours, when the heat commenced, and continued about seven hours, and was seldom followed by perspiration. The next day there was a lighter paroxysm, which usually commenced at twelve o'clock, and ceased about the same time in the evening, as the heavier one on the day preceding. The paroxysms continued to occur thus alternately with but little variation for the space of twenty-three days, notwithstanding my unceasing efforts to arrest them by the administration of a number of remedies.

On the twelfth of December, the following symptoms were present:—chill commenced at nine o'clock in the morning, and lasted four hours, attended with a great deal of shivering and trembling; raging thirst before the chill, and during the chill and heat; vomiting of whatever was taken into the stomach, and of bile, with distressing pain in the epigastrium; distracting headache during the heat; fever ceased about eight o'clock in the evening, and was followed by inconsiderable perspiration. Eup. p. 1, in water, a teaspoonful every hour in the apyrexia, cured the case, without the recurrence of another paroxysm.

CASE 2. Mrs. B. R. M——, living near the Schuylkill river, of bilious diathesis. A case of tertian ague. Chill at nine o'clock in the morning, which lasted an hour and a half; thirst in the night before the chill; raging thirst during the chill and heat; violent headache throughout the paroxysm; some perspiration; retching and vomiting during the chill, immediately after drinking; vomiting of bile. Eup. per. 1, five drops in as many teaspoonfuls of water, of which she took a teaspoonful every two hours on the alternate day. Early on the morning of the expected chill, eup. per. tinct. gtt. iv. in eight teaspoonfuls of water, a teaspoonful every hour. The paroxysm did not return. This patient had been subject to frequent attacks of intermittent fever for several years, and had always suppressed them with sulph. of quinine, but since the above attack, now a period of nearly four years, she has had no return of the disease.

CASE 3. M. P——, a girl of 14 years of age, living in the neighbourhood of Fairmount. Tertian intermittent fever. Thirst before the chill; became stretchy and looked pale at nine o'clock in the morning; felt cold and chilly, but did not shake; walked about the house crouched up; was very thirsty during the chill and heat, but took only a little sup of water at a time; headache and trembling during the heat, the coldness lasted an hour, and the heat about two hours; followed by very little perspiration. Eup. per. tinct. a few drops in water; dose, a teaspoonful every three hours. Cured.

CASE 4. A. P——, sister to the last patient, and living in the same house. At eight o'clock in the morning was attacked with pain above the right ilium, thirst and a disposition to yawn; fingers became stiff, with slight coldness; upon taking a drink of water, shuddering commenced immediately; chill lasted two hours and a half; headache, backache, and thirst during the chill; nausea as the chill was going off; the the headache was increased, but the thirst was diminished during the heat; sensation of great weakness during the fever, so much so, that she could not raise her head from the pillow; trembling in the back, with faintness from motion, during the fever. The fever terminated by moderate perspiration during sleep in the evening. She felt pain in her bones early in the morning before the attack. Eup. per. tinct. in water, a teaspoonful every three hours. Had but the one paroxysm.

CASE 5. T. R——, had tertian ague, for two weeks before I saw him. Sickly, sallow countenance; chill at eight o'clock in the morning; thirst throughout the night previous to the chill; thirst during the chill and heat, and vomiting immediately after each draught of water; vomiting of bile at the close of the hot stage, which was followed by inconsiderable perspiration. Eup. per. tinct. in water, a teaspoonful every three hours. (*Williamson.*)

"This herb, (Eupatorium perfoliatum,*) it is known, derived its domestic name of boneset, from its prompt manner of relieving pains in the limbs, and general muscular system, which attended a peculiar form of febrile disease, which prevailed many years ago in the northern parts of America. It was this fact, together with the knowledge of the remarkable combination of properties possessed by it, which led to the suggestion of its employment in epidemic influenza; and nothing could be more marked and satisfactory than the prompt manner in which it answered the expectations, which had been formed of it in this respect. The pain in the back and limbs, and the lassitude of the general muscular system, subsided so soon as the system was placed under its influence; its immediate and salutary operation in this way at once prominently exhibiting its great value in the treatment of disease. But its curative agency was not confined to this effect alone; for blended with this prompt action on the nervous system—for we can in no other way account for its speedy removal of the pains, and the general muscular prostration, except by referring its operation to the nervous system,—the Eupatorium perfoliatum united in its operation, other qualities, each one eminently adapted to fulfil some important indication in the treatment of the disease in question. Among the first of these we shall name its diaphoretic powers. The sudorific influence of this herb, is of that peculiar character which eminently fitted it for employment under the circumstances. For, in this disease, the skin was not unfrequently imbued with perspiration. But, probably, from a peculiar condition of the cutaneous surface, the sweating was of a morbid character, a sort of passive excretion, resulting apparently from a lax condition of the skin, which was always under such circumstances pale, and morbidly sensitive. This state of the cutaneous surface, particularly its morbid sensitiveness,

* American Jour. of Med. Sci., April 1844, p. 364.

in no small number of cases, constituted a curious, and not a little distressing, attendant on the disease.

The Eupatorium perfoliatum not only induced a healthy and free perspiratory discharge, but promptly altered the condition of the skin, restoring its natural hue, and rendering its texture firm and healthy; and the unpleasant alternations of chilliness with flushes of heat were replaced by an agreeable glow of the general surface. So soon as this diaphoresis was induced, together with the relief already mentioned as occurring, the disposition to cough subsided and there was an immediate amelioration of all the pulmonary symptoms. The subsidence of the cough, the renewal of the dyspnœa, and that painful irritation of the pulmonary organs, which in many cases seem to have extended to the remotest air vesicles of the lungs, were more directly due to the medicine administered after the method adopted by us, becoming a prompt and efficacious expectorant. Indeed, we know of no article or combination to be preferred to it as an expectorant in the disease under consideration. Together with the properties already mentioned, this medicine has further proved itself sufficiently aperient for the treatment of most cases of epidemic influenza. After the commencement of the treatment it was rarely found necessary to use any other cathartic, and not then, except in those cases in which the constipation of the bowels had been persistent, or where the head was unusually affected."

"Its tonic property is the remaining one which we shall point out, as particularly adapting this medicine to the treatment of certain cases of epidemic influenza. It certainly is a great desideratum, in the management of this disease, in aged subjects, where there is such a tendency to prostration long before any impression is made on the violence of the attack, to have a remedy which, with due evacuant powers adequate to the removal of all the symptoms, unites a tonic influence sufficient to support the general strength, and to maintain at the same time the integrity of the circulatory functions. The admirable association of its tonic with its other properties, creates in the Eupatorium perfoliatum such an agent, and endows it with an advantage over all articles or combinations, in the management of the disease under these circumstances. Indeed, when the disease was treated from the first with this medicine, the cold infusion alternated with the warm, according to the circumstances of the case, and the amount of prostration present—no case occurred where more decided stimulants or tonics were required; and we are convinced that the former preparation of this herb is the very best article of this class, not only to prevent, but to overcome when existing, the prostration so frequently supervening upon this disease in old persons. Nor were its salutary powers in this way confined alone to the aged. It has never, we believe, been noticed before,—and hence whether it is universally the case or not we have no means of judging,—but it is certain that the coloured population with us suffered in a peculiar manner from this disease. In almost every case from its very commencement, it assumed a marked and curiously asthenic character; yet upon the whole it was not more formidable, nor more difficult of management, than the same disorder in the white subjects."

"In these cases it seemed to expend its force upon the nervous system, producing a dispondency of mind, a depression of the vascular, and a prostration of the muscular systems, wholly disproportioned to all the other symptoms. It was no unusual occurrence, after a negro had staggered into the office as though he were intoxicated, and stated his case with a gloomy presentiment of evil, to find upon examination a prostration of the pulse really startling, while the pulmonary symptoms were trifling; and the bowels were free from the morbid contamination; in fact, the pain in the back and limbs, the remarkable and extreme lassitude of the muscular system, and the uneasiness about the head, being the only symptoms for which he sought relief. It was surprising how soon a few doses of the infusion of boneset, administered solely with a view to secure its tonic and aperient effects, would remove this state of things. There is yet another class of cases, to which this property of the herb, from its peculiar association, render it particularly applicable. The disease occurring in the habitually inebriate, induces a train of morbid effects in the highest degree embarrassing, and for the treatment of which we found nothing so salutary as its cold infusion, combined with the tincture or infusion of hops, according as the nature of the case required sedation."

"*Manner of administration.*—In the severest cases, where it is determined to treat the disease with the herb alone, the patient, after being covered in bed, was induced to swallow a wine-glassfull of the infusion, prepared by infusing an ounce of the dried leaves in a pint of boiling water, warm, every half hour. After the fourth or fifth dose, considerable nausea, sometimes vomiting, with free diaphoresis ensued, and there was an immediate amelioration of all the symptoms. Along with the nausea free expectoration commenced; and after the former symptom had subsided, the patient was freed from every annoyance, and remained in every respect comfortable. Sufficient to keep up the impression on the system, the infusion was now given only every third or fourth hour in the same dose. The bowels were generally opened in about six hours after the commencement of the treatment, and afterwards continued in a lax condition. Towards the evening the second day, and particularly if the patient had been guilty of imprudent exposure, the symptoms frequently returned, and it was necessary to repeat the course adopted at first. But generally the medicine, continued as directed, kept the symptoms completely in check, and the patient was out on the fourth day."

"The treatment of the disease in old persons, or in other cases where there was a marked tendency to prostration, was commenced in the same manner. As soon as the effects already mentioned as occurring were induced, the cold substituted for the warm infusion was directed in the same dose every second hour, to be continued, gradually lessening the period throughout the disease, unless the violent symptoms returned, when it was to be discontinued until the same course was repeated with the warm infusion, and then resumed."

"From the foregoing exposition of the properties and mode of action of the Eupatorium perfoliatum, we feel convinced that it will be awarded, that its introduction is an acquisition of some value to the therapeutical means of managing the curious disease under consideration. Not the least of our reasons for believing so, is, that while it allows the patient treated by it to pass out of the disease as speedily and as perfectly as any other remedy, or course of treatment, it leaves him with less impairment of his general health, and causes fewer interruptions to the natural healthy functions of the body. In short, the universality of the disease, when it prevails, finds an exact counterpart in the cheapness, as well as the simplicity of the remedy." *J. F. Pebbles, M. D.*

KALMIA LATIFOLIA.

BY C. HERING, M. D.

Vulgo. Laurel; Mountain Laurel; Broad-leaved Laurel; Lambkill; Ivy Bush; Spoonwood; Calico Bush.

Nat. Ord. Bicornes. *Linn.*
Rhododendra. *Juss.*

Class. Decandria.

Order. Monogynia.

The genus is called Kalmia, in honour of Peter Kalm, a Sweedish Botanist.

GEN. CHAR. *Calyx* five-parted, persistent, with oval acute segments.

Corolla salver-form, with ten horns beneath, and ten corresponding cavities within.

Capsule five-celled, many seeded.

SPEC. CHAR. Leaves petioled, inserted on the sides and extremities of the branches, scattered, and in threes; oval, acute, entire, coriaceous, smooth on both sides, under side the palest; corymbs terminal, siscid and pubescent, simple or compound, with opposite branches and made up of slender peduncles, supported at base by ovate acuminate bractes.

Flowers in the latter end of May.

Fruit mature in the beginning of September.

An evergreen shrub, from three to twelve feet high, and grows on shaded rocky hills.

Flowers rose red, sometimes white.

The corolla is monopetalous, with a cylindrical tube, a spreading disk, and an erect five-cleft margin.

The stamens proceed from the base of the corolla, and bend outwardly like a hoop, so as to bury their anthers in the little cells of the corolla, until the fecundating power of the pollen is perfect, when they spring up and strike against the stigma.

The germ is globular; style longer than the corolla, and declined; stigma obtuse.

The capsule is roundish, depressed, five-celled, and five-valved.

When chemically examined the leaves are found to contain vegetable mucus, tannin and resin.

Kalmia latifolia is destined to become a very important remedy in the treatment of acute, and also of chronic diseases.

As Ledum inhabits the marshy meadows among the mountains of Europe, and as Rhododendron, beautifies the mountain plains of Asia, with its golden blossoms, so Kalmia frequently extends itself along both banks of the narrow stony valleys of the brooks and small streams of North America, and enlivens them with its broad evergreen leaves; and in May it suddenly spreads a rose coloured carpet over the face of nature, which excites the admiration even of those who are accustomed to the magnificence of tropical plants. Rhododendron thrives in the region of storms and mountains, and Ledum draws its nourishment from the ponds of elevated regions, while Kalmia flourishes in the mists arising from the valleys. All three inhabit northern climates. They correspond to the great family of diseases, which we comprise under the collective names of rheumatism and gout; particularly to that class, which belongs to the north, and which is decidedly distinct from that of the south, and of the tropics. They also correspond to the intermittent and remittent fevers, and especially those of a long protracted gastric-nervous character.

No medicine in the whole Materia Medica, has such control over the pulse as kalmia, except digitalis. Aconite and tartar emetic, approximate to it; but a remedy can only diminish the activity of the heart *favourably*, when it corresponds to the totality of the symptoms. In diseases of the heart, which alternate with rheumatism or have originated in rheumatic attacks, kalmia must become most important. It will be of great service to the veterinarian. The other characteristics of this medicine are seen by the pathogenesis.

Our attention is called to the action of this plant; first, by the poisoning of young domestic animals, and the sickening of the older ones from eating the leaves; secondly, by the diseases which are caused by the honey gathered by the bees from its blossoms; thirdly, by the illness caused by eating the pheasant's nourished by the fruit and green leaves during the winter months; and fourthly, by the Indians making use of it to commit suicide.

The Indians kill themselves with an infusion of the leaves. *Barton.*

From my own experience I am not disposed to think very highly of the narcotic power of the kalmia. I have repeatedly chewed and swallowed a green leaf of the largest size, without perceiving the least effect in consequence. *Bigelow.*

It must be used with great care when externally applied, as the decoction has occasioned disagreeable subsultus, startings and convulsions. *Barton.*

The leaves are poisonous to some animals, and food for others. *Kalm.*

It is food for deer, goats, partridges and pheasants. *U. S. Dispensatory.*

Deer feed on its green leaves with impunity. *Catesby.*

The leaves of kalmia are food for stags, and if they be shot in winter their bowels are found filled with them. *Bigelow.*

Persons who have eaten the flesh of stags that have fed on the leaves of kalmia, have not felt the least indisposition from it. *Bigelow.*

If the bowels of deer which have fed on the leaves be given to dogs, they become quite stupid, and as it were intoxicated; and often become so sick as to appear to be at the point of death. *Bigelow.*

It is fatal to young animals. *Bigelow.*

When cattle and sheep, by severe winters deprived of better food, feed on the leaves of this plant, a great many of them die annually. *Catesby.*

When sheep eat kalmia leaves, they are attacked with vomiting, bleeding at the nose, and vertigo. *U.*

When sheep eat the leaves, they either die immediately, or become very sick, and recover with great difficulty. The young and more tender of them are killed by a small portion, but the older and more hardy ones can bear a stronger dose. *Kalm.*

It produces the same noxious effect on calves; they either die or recover with great difficulty. *Kalm.*

Some calves, after eating of the leaves in 1748, became very sick, swelled, frothed at the mouth, and could scarcely stand; they were cured, however, by giving them gun-powder and other remedies. *Kalm.*

A few drops of the tincture poured upon the body of a large and vigorous rattlesnake, killed it in a very short time. *Barton.*

Horses, oxen and cows are made very sick by eating the leaves, but do not die. *Bigelow.*

Gastric disorders and delirium have been caused by eating the honey gathered from the flowers. *Barton.*

The infusion is used in dysentery. *U.*

* A diarrhœa which returned every eight weeks, was cured by a decoction of one ounce of the leaves with eight ounces of water, and boiled down one-half. *Thomas.*

* Kalmia has been used with much benefit in the cure of syphilis. *U. S. D.*

An ointment made of the powdered leaves has been recommended in tinea capitis, and some other cutaneous affections. *Bigelow.*

I have seen an eruption, very much resembling psora, removed by it. *Bigelow.*

Externally applied in the shape of ointment or decoction, the leaves have been found useful in tinea capitis, psora, herpes, and other cutaneous affections. *U. S. D.*

The powdered leaves have been used with success by an empiric, in certain fevers. *Barton.*

14

Kalmia has the remarkable peculiarity of depressing the pulse when given in large doses. *U.*

The pulse reduced to forty strokes in a minute, with great weakness in the arms and calves of the legs, and vertigo, on every attempt to move; in a recumbent posture, the mental faculties and memory are perfect. *U.*

Two cases of poisoning, which resulted from eating a pheasant, in the craw of which laurel leaves were found.

1. Half an hour after eating, nausea with entire loss of sight; continual retching and violent pain in the crown of the head, which extends down in the direction of the cervicle vertebræ; coldness of the extremities, and imperceptible pulse; when the pulse reappeared it beat only forty strokes in a minute.

2. A peculiar noise while breathing, like that caused by spasmodic affections of the glottis. Paleness of the face. Excessive nausea, with dimness before the eyes. Violent pain down the back. Coldness of the extremities, with a very feeble pulse, of forty strokes in a minute. *Shoemaker.*

Kalmia is useful in acute and chronic diseases of the lungs. *U.*

The names of the provers are attached to their symptoms as well as the number of the attenuations taken.

Those marked *a*, *b*, *c*, etc., represent persons under Mr. Behlert's care, whose temperaments are carefully described in his report.

Those extracts marked *U.*, are taken from an American author, to me unknown.

In making the trials, (as is my custom,) the low and high dilutions were both employed in the same persons, where it was practicable; and he who does not or will not see the resemblance of the symptoms severally produced by them, is to be pitied; but to perceive the difference, requires practice and close investigation.

MENTAL.—1. Irritable disposition of the mind towards evening, which continues next morning. (3*d.* *Reichhelm.*)

Indisposition to move, with aversion to exercise. (2*d.* *E. Clark.*)

SLEEP.—Restlessness, frequent turning. (2*d.* *E. Clark.*)

Getting up and walking, while asleep. (2*d.* *E. Clark.*)

5. Talking in sleep. (2*d.* *E. Clark.*)

Unpleasant dreams. (2*d.* *E. Clark.*)

Fantastic dreams. (30*th.* *Haeseler.*)

FEVER.—Cold and shivering on two successive days. (2*d.* *E. Clark.*)

HEAD.—Vertigo and headache. *Puihn.*

10. Vertigo, (from 30 drops of the infusion, six times a day.) *Thomas.*

Vertigo, with some nausea, attended with pains in the head and limbs. (30*th.* *Kummer.*)

Nausea in the evening, followed by some dulness and aching in the head. (The second day. 30*th.* *Kummer.*)

Vertigo while stooping and looking downwards. (From 8 until 9 o'clock in the morning, and from 3 until 6 o'clock in the evening. 30*th.* *Behlert.*)

Dulness in the head. (First day. 1*st.* *Kummer.*)

15. Dulness in the head in the evening. (3*d.* *Kummer.*)

Dulness in the head until evening, which continues slightly early the next morning. (3*d.* *Kummer.*)

Heaviness in the head for a short time on the right side, but towards evening the same sensation, very severe on the left side. (1*st.* *Kummer.*)

Heat in the head, on the morning of the fifth day. (3*d.* *Reichhelm.*)

A shock towards the occiput from the back of the neck with heat. (30*th.* *Behlert. a.*)

20. A momentary shivering without coldness, about 10 o'clock in the evening in bed, which seems to pass from the top of the head to the neck under the scalp, attend-

ed with a cracking noise, and at the same time alarm without palpitation of the heart; a sensation as if the body were surcharged with electricity. This sensation was repeated four times in the course of half an hour, and the whole ended with the sound of a horn before the ears. (3*d*. *Reichhelm.*)

Headache internally, with the sensation, when turning, of something loose in the head, diagonally across the top of it. (30*th*. *Behlert. b.*)

Dull pain around the back part of the head, with frequent sharp, darting pain in the right side of the head. (2*d*. *E. Clark.*)

Pain in the head when awaking in the morning, and in the evening. (2*d*. *E. Clark.*)

Pain in the top of the head as if bound closely with a cord. (2*d*. *E. Clark.*)

25. Strong pain in the temples and forehead. (2*d*. *E. Clark.*)

Pain in the forehead every morning on awaking. (30*th*. *Behlert. c.*)

Pain in the forehead on rising, which increases afterwards. (30*th*. *Behlert. f.*)

Pain across the forehead over the eyes. (30*th*. *Behlert. c.*)

Rending pain across the forehead. (30*th*. *Behlert. d.*)

30. Pressing pain in the forehead especially in the right side. (First day. 3*d*. *Reichhelm.*)

Pain in the forehead in the evening. (30*th*. *Behlert. a.*)

Pressing in the forehead, late in the evening. (3*d*. *Reichhelm.*)

Pain in the forehead and over the eyes in the evening; it seems to move backwards and down the neck outwardly on both sides, then disappears, and is followed by pain in the left shoulder. (30*th*. *Behlert. a.*)

The pain in the forehead is sometimes followed by rending in the bones of the right or left side of the face, or on the top of the head. (30*th*. *Behlert. c.*)

35. Slight aching in the forehead, which some times

shoots downwards to the eye-teeth, and at one time is easier in the forehead, at another in the teeth. (30*th*. *Behlert.* *a.*)

Pains in the forehead every day, which extends to the roots of one of the upper molar teeth of the right side. (30*th*. *Behlert.* *a.*)

Severe pressing in the temples, and on both sides of the neck. (30*th*. *Kummer.*)

Acute pain in the left temple, which is very much increased by going up stairs. (2*d*. *Williamson.*)

Rending in the forehead and in the head, on rising from bed, succeeded by rending in the bones of the hips and lower extremities, down to the feet. (30*th*. *Behlert.* *a.*)

40. Rending in the head and neck. (30*th*. *Behlert.* *a.*)

Rending in the head. (30*th*. *Behlert.* *c.*)

Rending in the left side of the forehead, which extends into the temple. (30*th*. *Behlert.* *c.*)

Strong pressure in the right temple. (The 3d day. 1*st*. *Kummer.*)

Rending in the right temple, passing downwards. (30*th*. *Behlert.* *c.*)

45. Severe headache at noon of the second day; it is most severe in the right side. (1*st*. *Kummer.*)

Pulsating pain in forehead. (30*th*. *Behlert.* *b.*)

Pain and throbbing in the whole of the left side of the head, with stitches in the left ear, and behind the right. (30*th*. *Kummer.*)

The drawing in the head and eyes is worse towards evening, and in the open air. (*Kummer.*)

EYES.—50. Glimmering before the eyes, exactly in the point of vision, so that it is almost impossible to distinguish the words while reading; it seems as if small points were continually moving before the eyes. This continues half an hour. (About 3 o'clock in the afternoon of the second day. 30*th*. *Kummer.*)

Glimmering before the eyes while looking downwards, with belching of wind, and some nausea. (In the morning about eight or nine o'clock. 30*th*. *Behlert.*)

Cloudiness before the eyes. (The third day. 1*st.* *Kummer.*)

Itching of the eyes, and stinging when rubbed. (2*d.* *E. Clark.*)

Pain in the eyes which makes it painful to turn them. (2*d.* *E. Clark.*)

55. Sensation of stiffness in the muscles around the eyes, and of the eyelids. (2*d.* *E. Clark.*)

Pain in the right eye. (1*st.* *Kummer.*)

Strong pressing in the right eye, in the evening. (1*st.* *Kummer.*)

Pressing in the eyes, attended by pains in the arms and hands, in the lower extremities down to the feet, and sometimes in the right side of the abdomen. (30*th.* *Kummer.*)

A sensation of pressing, above the right eye. (About noon of the 3d day. 3*d.* *Reichhelm.*)

60. Pressing pain about the eyes. (The 5th day. 3*d.* *Reichhelm.*)

Pressing in the eyes in the afternoon. (3*d.* *Reichhelm.*)

Acute stitches in the eyes, towards evening of the second day. (1*st.* *Kummer.*)

Acute stitches in the right eye, in the morning of the second day. (1*st.* *Kummer.*)

Stitches and violent pressing in the right eye, the eyes feel dim and weak. (The third day. 1*st.* *Kummer.*)

65. Stitches under the left eye. (30*th.* *Kummer.*)

Itching in the eyes. (1*st.* *Kummer.*)

Itching and burning in the left eye. (In the afternoon of the fifth day. (3*d.* *Reichhelm.*)

Burning with pressing in the eyes, particularly in the left one. (The fifth day. 3*d.* *Reichhelm.*)

Inflammation of the left eye in the morning, with a burning jerking pain, till near noon, when the pain becomes more tolerable, and scarcely perceptible. (The sixth day. 3*d.* *Reichhelm.*)

EARS.—70. Severe stitches in the right ear, in the night of the second day. (1*st.* *Kummer.*)

Severe stitches in the ears at 4 o'clock, P. M., followed by pain in the arms. (30*th*. *Kummer.*)

Pain the right ear, on the right side of the head, and in the leg. (30*th*. *Kummer.*)

Excessive tingling in the ears. (In the afternoon of the fourth day. 3*d*. *Reichhelm.*)

NOSE.—Continued pressing in the ridge of the nose, with repeated sneezing. (The second day. 3*d*. *Reichhelm.*)

75. Tickling in the nose. (30*th*. *Behlert*. *a.*)

Fluent coryza with frequent sneezing, and perceptibly increased sense of smell. (30*th*. *Haeseler.*)

Tickling in the nose like that which precedes coryza. (30*th*. *Behlert*. *d.*)

The nose is sometimes obstructed, particularly in the evening. (30*th*. *Behlert*. *d.*)

FACE.—Pressing pain in the right side of the face, between the eye and the nose, in the afternoon. (3*d*. *Reichhelm.*)

80. Itching in the face at night. (30*th*. *Behlert*. *a.*)

Stinging in the bones of the jaws. (30*th*. *Behlert*. *a.*)

TEETH.—Short pains in the teeth of the right side, in the evening of the third day. (1*st*. *Kummer.*)

Pain in the upper teeth. (30*th*. *Kummer.*)

Severe pressing in the molar teeth after 10 o'clock in the evening, which continues several hours. (3*d*. *Reichhelm.*)

85. Dull pain in the incisor and eye-teeth. (3*d*. *Reichhelm.*)

MOUTH.—Stiches in the tongue. (30*th*. *Kummer.*)

Tongue white and dry. (2*d*. *E. Clark.*)

Lips swollen, dry and stiff, in the morning. (2*d*. *E. Clark.*)

Tingling in the salivary glands, immediately after eating, attended with a sensation of fermentation in the œsophagus, and copious salivation. (30*th*. *Haeseler.*)

90. Dry skin and cracked lips. (30*th*. *Haeseler.*)

Inflammation of the sublingual glands. (*W. Link.*)

Acrid, bitter taste in the mouth. *U.*

THROAT.—Continual rising of a slippery mucus in the throat, with tickling in the larynx. (30*th. Haeseler.*)

Difficult deglutition. (30*th. Kummer.*)

Dryness of the throat, which renders deglutition difficult. Thirsty. (2*d. E. Clark.*)

95. Scraping in the throat. (30*th. Behlert. a.*)

Scraping in the throat, which excites a cough day and night. (30*th. Behlert. c.*)

Pressing in the throat and nausea, with stitches in the eyes. (30*th. Kummer.*)

Sensation of rawness and scraping in the throat, which is painful while swallowing, and is attended by throbbing in the left tonsil. (30*th. Behlert.*)

STOMACH.—Pressing in the scrobiculus cordis, which is relieved by sitting erect, but is aggravated by sitting in a crooked position. (30*th. Haeseler.*)

100. Nausea, with headache. (30*th. Behlert. a.*)

ABDOMEN.—Pain in the right side of the abdomen followed by a pain in the gluteus muscle. (30*th. Kummer.*)

A sensation of weakness in the abdomen, rising up into the throat. When violent, it is sometimes relieved by eructations, but returns immediately. (30*th. Behlert. a.*)

Occasional pain across the abdomen. (2*d. E. Clark.*)

Pressing in the right side. (30*th. Behlert. a.*)

105. Pain in the right side, in the region of the liver. (2*d. E. Clark.*)

BOWELS.—No stool the first day. (3*d. Reichhelm.*)

Scanty stool. (The morning of the third day. 3*d. Reichhelm.*)

Looseness of the bowels at noon. After the stool in the morning. (3*d. Reichhelm.*)

Stools less frequent. (The third day. 3*d. Reichhelm.*)

110. A soft stool early in the morning, followed by

a diarrhœa, which lasted two hours, and another soft stool the same forenoon. (The fourth day. 3*d*. *Reichhelm.*)

Inclination to go to stool. (The forenoon of the fourth day. 3*d*. *Reichhelm.*)

Two soft stools, and an evacuation of wind. (The forenoon of the fifth day. 3*d*. *Reichhelm.*)

Momentary nausea, with shifting of flatus in the afternoon while riding, followed by a stool, with cutting pain in the bowels. (The third day, after repeated doses. 3*d*. *Reichhelm.*)

Easily discharged, pappy stool, with pressing in the rectum. (30*th*. *Haeseler.*)

URINE.—115. Strong desire to urinate. (The ninth day. 3*d*. *Reichhelm.*)

Frequent discharges of yellow urine, in increased quantity. (30*th*. *Haeseler.*)

SEXUAL.—The menses appear eight days too early. (The fourth day. 30*th*. *Behlert. c.*)

The menses make their appearance fourteen days too late. (30*th*. *Behlert. c.*)

Painful menstruation. (2*d*. *E. Clark.*)

120. Suppression of the menses. (2*d*. *E. Clark.*)

Postponement of the menses. (2*d*. *E. Clark.*)

Pain in the loins, back, and anterior part of the thighs during menstruation. (2*d*. *E. Clark.*)

Yellowish leucorrhœa in the morning, eight days after the appearance of the menses. (Three weeks after the exhibition of kalmia. 30*th*. *Behlert. a.*)

The symptoms are more prominent during the leucorrhœa. (30*th*. *Behlert. a.*)

LARYNX.—125. Cough excited, by scraping in the wind-pipe. (30*th*. *Behlert. d.*)

Cough, with easy expectoration of a gray, smooth unctuous matter, which has a putrid, saltish taste. (30*th*. *Haeseler.*)

CHEST.—Oppression and shortness of breath, which obliges him to breath quickly, involuntarily. (30*th*. *Haeseler.*)

Oppression of the chest. After the fifth dose, every fourth day. (30*th.* *Kummer.*)

Oppression of the chest, difficulty of breathing, dulness of the head, and nausea. (30*th.* *Kummer.*)

130. Sensation in the chest, as if strained by lifting. (2*d.* *E. Clark.*)

Stitches in the lower part of the chest. (30*th.* *Behlert. a.*)

Oppression of the chest, with the sensation of swelling in the throat. (*W. Link.*)

Palpitation of the heart. (*W. Link.*)

TRUNK.—Violent pressure in the right side of the neck, and at the same time in the left foot. (1*st.* *Kummer.*)

135. Drawing and sticking in the left side of the neck, in the afternoon which continues eight hours. (3*d.* *Reichhelm.*)

Acute stitches and itching on the left side of the neck at night. (30*th.* *Behlert.*)

Stitches under the left arm. (30*th.* *Kummer.*)

A sensation as if the spinal column would break with an anterior convexity. (30*th.* *Haeseler.*)

Sharp pain in the three superior dorsal vertebræ, extending through the shoulder blades. (2*d.* *E. Clark.*)

140. Constant pain in the spine, sometimes worse in the lumbar region, with great heat and burning. (2*d.* *E. Clark.*)

Pressing below the left shoulder, in the evening. (Second day. 3*d.* *Reichhelm.*)

Pain in the shoulder blades. (2*d.* *E. Clark.*)

Sticking pain in the lower part of the left shoulder blade, the night after the third day. (1*st.* *Kummer.*)

Aching pain across the loins, worse in the evening. (2*d.* *Williamson.*)

145. Paralytic pain in the small of the back, at ten o'clock at night in bed, with continued dulness and pain in the head. (The second day. 3*d.* *Reichhelm.*)

Lameness in the small of the back, in the evening in bed. (The third day. 3*d.* *Reichhelm.*)

UPPER EXTREMITIES.—Rending in the right shoulder and down the arm. (30*th*. *Behlert. c.*)

Rending in the shoulder joint. (30*th*. *Behlert. a.*)

Drawing pain on the inner side of the left arm, of short duration. (The third day. 1*st*. *Kummer.*)

Pain in the right arm. (1*st*. *Kummer.*)

150. Frequent strong cracking in the joints of the elbows, in the afternoon. (3*d*. *Reichhelm.*)

Rending from the left elbow, down the arm to the index figer, which is flexed in a jerking manner. (30*th*. *Behlert. f.*)

Cramp-like pain, from the elbow down to the middle of the forearm. (30*th*. *Behlert. c.*)

Rending from the knuckle of the little finger of the right hand, up to the elbow. (30*th*. *Behlert. f.*)

Repeated stitches in the hands. (30*th*. *Behlert. a.*)

155. Pains in the right hand. (30*th*. *Behlert. f.*)

Pains in the left hand, particularly in the palm close to the wrist. (After the sixth dose. 30*th*. *Kummer.*)

A sensation like paralysis in the right hand. (After six doses. 30*th*. *Kummer.*)

Pain in the left wrist, so that the hand seems palsied. (1*st*. *Kummer.*)

Pain in all the fingers of the left hand at the same time. (The third day. 1*st*. *Kummer.*)

LOWER EXTREMITIES.—160. Stitches suddenly attacking the hip bones of the right side, in the evening. (30*th*. *Behlert. a.*)

Stiches on the lower part of the knee, outside, in the evening. (30*th*. *Behlert. a.*)

Itching in the bend of the right knee, in the afternoon of the ninth day. (3*d*. *Reichhelm.*)

Pains in the left knee and foot, and also in the right foot, repeatedly. (Third day. 30*th*. *Kummer.*)

Numbness in the shins, in the afternoon. (3*d*. *Reichhelm.*)

165. A peculiar pain along the outside of the left leg, which is very frequently repeated. (30*th*. *Kummer.*)

Pain in the left foot. (1*st.* *Kummer.*)

Great weariness in the evening, particularly in the extremities, so that it is nearly impossible to go up stairs. (2*d.* *E. Clark.*)

Numbness of the limbs, as if asleep. (2*d.* *E. Clark.*)

Violent pain in the left foot. (The tenth day. 1*st.* *Kummer.*)

170. Pain in the left foot. (After the fifth dose. 30*th.* *Kummer.*)

Aching in the tarsal bones of the right foot. (30*th.* *Behlert. f.*)

Sticking in the soles of the feet. (30*th.* *Behlert. a.*)

Stinging in the toes. (30*th.* *Behlert. c.*)

Stinging in the great toe of the left foot. (30*th.* *Behlert. c.*)

175. Pain in the left arm above the elbow, and soon afterwards between the elbow and the hand; frequently alternating between the two places, during one hour, and followed by pain in both legs below the knees, which extends to the feet. (1*st.* *Kummer.*)

Brief pains in the left elbow, arm, and knee, in the morning, and in both arms in the afternoon; while lying it is not observed. (The third day. 30*th.* *Kummer.*)

Pain in the bend of the left knee, which is immediately followed by very severe, frequent but brief pain in the left index finger, and afterwards in the right foot. (1*st.* *Kummer.*)

Pain in the right shoulder and in the left arm, particularly in the elbow, and in both lower extremities, especially in the knees. (30*th.* *Kummer.*)

Pain in the left arm and in both legs, in the evening. (30*th.* *Kummer.*)

180. Pressing pain in the left shin, and in the muscles of the left arm, accompanied with the same kind of pain in the right foot. (1*st.* *Kummer.*)

Pressing in the left shin, at eight o'clock in the

morning, and in the left shoulder at ten o'clock in the morning. (30*th*. *Kummer.*)

Pressing in the left shin and shoulder, and also in the left arm, followed by pressing in the right shoulder and arm. (30*th*. *Kummer.*)

Pain in the right arm, and rending in the left leg, while at rest, which disappears on rising. It extends through the whole of the left side and arm. (30*th*. *Behlert. c.*)

Rending in the right shoulder, in the left arm, in the right under-jaw bone, and in the flesh of the whole of the left leg downwards. (30*th*. *Behlert. c.*)

185. Slight aching in the left hand and fingers, and in the posterior part of the left leg, towards the heel, with jerking in the heel. (30*th*. *Behlert. a.*)

Sticking pain in the right index finger, in the evening, which is soon followed by a severe pain in the hollow of the right knee and in the calf of the leg, attended by difficulty of breathing. (After six doses. 30*th*. *Kummer.*)

Frequent pains here and there in the limbs, continually changing from one place to another, for ten days, during the exhibition of a few globules every second day. They lasted three weeks after the discontinuance of the medicine. (1*st*. *Kummer.*)

Frequent pains in the muscles of the extremities, and also in the head, with dulness, vertigo, and some nausea. (30*th*. *Kummer.*)

Sprain-like pain at times in the feet and hands. (30*th*. *Kummer.*)

190. A red spot, about the size of a pea, appeared on the outside of the left leg, a little below the knee, which itched excessively and was followed by a burning pain. This was succeeded by a second on the outside of the leg close to the knee, with excessive itching. (From the afternoon of the sixth to the seventh day.) On the morning of the seventh day a small spot appeared on the right knee, also with some itching of short duration. (3*d*. *Reichhelm.*)

15

Red inflamed spots in different places on the body, which appear like the beginning of blood-boils, and continue for several weeks. (*Bute.*)

Pressing pains in the whole body, in one hour and a half after taking the third dose of six globules, which had been repeated every fourth day. (30*th.* *Kummer.*)

The pains are most severe while moving, and disappear while lying. (30*th.* *Kummer.*)

The symptoms subsided gradually and successively, having all disappeared on the sixth day. (*E. Clark.*)

LOBELIA.

BY JACOB JEANES, M. D.

LOBELIA. *Sex. Syst.* Pentandria, Monogynia.

Nat. Ord. Lobeliacea.

GEN. CH. *Calyx* five-cleft. *Corolla* irregular, five-parted, cleft on the upper side nearly to the base. *Anthers* united into a tube. *Stigma* two-lobed. *Capsule* inferior or semi-superior, two or three-celled, two-valved at the apex. *Torrey.*

"Father Plumier dedicated a genus of plants to Mathias de Lobel, or de L'Obel, author of a history of plants in 1576. The plant to which he originally applied the name of Lobelia, is now the scævola, of Linnæus. When this botanist was convinced by Jacquin, that, under the name of Lobelia, a vast number of plants, generically distinct from the original plant, were confounded with it, and that these plants were better known than the true Lobelia, by that name, he judged it proper to correct the error by retaining this name for them, and giving a new one to the genus of Plumier. This is the origin of the term Lobelia for the genus as it now stands." *Barton.*

The growing together of the anthers in a tube, has caused differences of opinion among botanists as to what place suits it in the Linnean system. Linnæus places it in syngenesia monogamia, while most modern botanists have removed it to the first order of the fifth class. Pursh and Barton agree in assigning it to monadelphia.

The lobelia forms a numerous family, containing about 160 species, of which 75 grow in America, 22 in New Holland, 32 in Africa, 12 in Asia, and 6 in Europe, whilst it is yet unknown to what countries the remaining species are indigenous.

Several species of lobelia have attracted attention as medicinal agents; but as the one at present of the greatest importance, we will first consider the

LOBELIA INFLATA.

Emetic Herb. Indian Tobacco.

"The Lobelia inflata is a biennial inelegant plant, about one foot, and from that to two feet high. The root is fibrous, yellowish-white, of an acrid taste, resembling that of tobacco. Stem upright, always solitary, angular, leafy, very pubescent, sometimes hirsute, and very much branched about mid-way. Branches axillary, shorter than the stem, which rises from six to ten inches above the top of the highest branches. The leaves are irregularly scattered and alternate, sometimes crowded, oval, generally sessile, with the margins unequally indented with tooth-like serratures. The flowers are numerous, situated on terminal leafy racemes, and supported on short axillary peduncles. The corolla is monopetalous and labiate; the lower lip three, and the upper two-toothed, is of a pale blue colour externally, and delicate violet within. The calix leaves are awl-shaped, and the length of the corolla. Seeds numerous, very small, and contained in egg-shaped inflated capsules, which have given rise to the specific appellation of the plant." *Barton.*

Samuel Thomson, who considered himself the discoverer of the medical properties of the Lobelia inflata, appears to have watched its growth with an almost paternal affection, and therefore the following extract from his account of the emetic herb, as he terms it, will not be without interest.*

"The emetic herb may be found in the first stages of its growth at all times through the summer, from the bigness of a six cent piece to that of a dollar, and larger,

* New Guide to Health, or Botanic Physician, page 43.

lying flat on the ground, in a round form, like a rose pressed flat, in order to bear the weight of snow which lays on it during the winter, and is subject to be winter-killed, like wheat. In the spring, it looks yellow and pale, like other things suffering from the wet and cold; but when the returning sun spreads forth its enlivening rays upon it, it lifts up its leaves, and shoots forth a stalk to the height of from twelve to fifteen inches, with a number of branches, carrying up its leaves with its growth. In July, it puts forth small, pale-blue blossoms, which are followed by small pods, about the size of a white bean, containing numerous very small seeds. This pod is an exact resemblance of the human stomach, having an inlet and an outlet higher than the middle; from the inlet it receives nourishment, and by the outlet discharges the seeds. It comes to maturity about the first of September, when the leaves and pods turn a little yellow; this is the best time to gather it. It is what is called by botanists, a biennial plant, or only of two years existence."

"This plant is common in all parts of this country. Wherever the land is fertile enough to yield support for its inhabitants, it is to be found. It is confined to no soil which is fit for cultivation, from the highest mountains to the lowest vallies. In hot and wet seasons, it is most plenty on dry and warm lands; in hot and dry seasons, on clayey and heavy land. When the season is cold, either wet or dry, it rarely makes its appearance; and if the summer and fall are very dry, the seed does not come up, and, of course, there will be very little to be found the next season. I have been in search of this herb from Boston to Canada, and was not able to collect more than two pounds; and in some seasons, I have not been able to collect any."

This is probably a very correct description of the growth of this plant in our Eastern States, and notwithstanding the peculiarities of expression, and the singular remark in relation to the pod, deserves to be copied, in the language of its author, for its exhibition of his loving watchfulness and close observation of his favorite plant, as well as for the real information it conveys.

It will be well to give Thomson's account of his discovery of the properties of the Lobelia inflata; he says: "Some time in the summer, after I was four years old, being out in the fields in search of the cows, I discovered a plant which had a singular branch and pods, that I had never before seen, and I had the curiosity to pick some of the pods and chew them; the taste and operation produced were so remarkable, that I never forgot it. I afterwards used to induce other boys to chew it, merely by way of sport to see them vomit. I tried this herb in this way for nearly twenty years, without knowing any thing of its medical virtues." "It had never occurred to me that it was of any value as medicine, until, when mowing in the field with a number of men one day, I cut a sprig of it, and gave to the man next to me, who eat it; when we had got to the end of the piece, which was about six rods, he said he believed what I had given him would kill him, for he never felt so in his life. I looked at him, and saw that he was in a most profuse perspiration, being wet all over as he could be; he trembled very much, and there was no more color in him than a corpse. I told him to go to the spring and drink some water; he attempted to go, and got as far as the wall, but was unable to get over it, and laid down on the ground and vomited several times. He said he thought he threw off his stomach two quarts. I then helped him into the house, and in about two hours he ate a very hearty dinner, and in the afternoon was able to do a good half day's labor. He afterwards told me that he never had any thing to do him so much good in his life; his appetite was remarkably good, and he felt better than he had for a long time." It afterwards became his most important remedy.

It is a customary remark of the writers on the Lobelia inflata, that it was employed as a remedy by the aborigines of this country; but no authority has been quoted for this assertion, which may therefore be viewed as groundless. Dr. Cutler first introduced this article to the attention of the medical profession. He had long suffered from asthma, when he was informed by Dr. Drury, of Marblehead, that he had been relieved of this complaint by the use of the tincture of the Lobelia inflata. He employed it, and was cured. For his case, see Appendix. This knowledge of the value of the Lobelia inflata, as a remedy in asthma, was most probably derived from the practice of Thomson in that neighborhood.

In support of this claim Thomson says, that, "In the fall of the year 1807, I introduced the use of the emetic herb tinctured in spirits, for the asthma and other complaints of the lungs, and cured several of the consumption. In 1808, I cured a woman in Newington of the asthma, who had not laid in her bed for six months. I gathered some of the young plants, not bigger than a dollar, bruised them, and tinctured them in spirits, gave her the tincture, and she lay in bed the first night. I showed her what it was, and how to prepare and use it; and by taking this and other things, according to my direction, she has enjoyed a comfortable state of health for twelve years, and has never been obliged to sit up one night since. The same fall I used it in Beverly and Salem ; and there can be no doubt but all the information concerning the value of this article was obtained from my practice."

A Charles Whitlaw tells, in the London Lancet, a queer story about hide bound cattle seeking and eating the Lobelia inflata, becoming salivated, and then getting well, and also that it is to him that the American practitioners are indebted for a knowledge of its medicinal properties. "When grass is scarce, it is eaten by cattle," but that it salivates them is yet to be proved, and it is a strange circumstance that no acknowledgment of their indebtedness to Charles Whitlaw should be made by American writers on the Lobelia inflata. I should not have noticed his remarks at all, had he not been quoted by Noack in his treatise.

Introduced into practice by a common man, who set himself in opposition to the customary modes of practice, the lobelia has met the fate of being represented by physicians as a medicine, which, from the violence of its effects, and the distressing nausea which it occasions, would never come into use for the common purposes of an emetic, while other emetics can be obtained; so that such a dread of its baneful effects have been instilled into the minds of physicians, that it has never been as much as tried by them as might have been expected. On the other hand, the followers of Thomson, whilst they admit that it is sometimes violent in its operation, deny that it is ever dangerous. The truth in this case, no doubt, lies between the two extremes. From the very limited number of deaths which have come to our knowledge, and can be fairly attributed to the Lobelia inflata, notwithstanding its extensive, and no doubt, rash employment by ignorant men, we must come to the conclusion that it is perhaps less dangerous and destructive than tartarized antimony, and many other of those substances which are in ordinary use for their emetic properties, would be if similarly employed.

Cutler states that the Lobelia inflata "operates as an emetic and then as a cathartic, its effects being much the same as those of the common emetics and cathartics;" but he does not confirm this statement by any cases. Thomson asserts that "as to its operating as a cathartic, I never knew it to have such an effect in all my practice." This assertion from one who must have employed it in thousands of cases, is entitled to attention, and I believe it will be found to be true in respect to the large emetic doses. But in doses of a few drops of the tincture, cathartic effects have been observed by several experimenters. Not doubting in the least the accuracy of the latter observations, I remain satisfied, from all the evidence I have been able to collect, that the large emetic doses rarely if ever purge, and that in this respect the operation of the Lobelia inflata differs very widely from that of ipecacuana and other emeto-cathartics.

In regard to the dose, there appears to be a singular agreement between Thomson and the physicians. He says, "Dr. Thatcher undertakes to make it appear that the fatal effects he tells about it producing," (in a fatal case treated by Thomson, for which he was tried for murder,) "was owing to the quantity given; and says, I administered a tea-spoonful of the powder; and when he comes to give directions for using it, says that from ten to twenty grains may be given with safety. It appears strange that different terms should produce such different effects in the operation of medicine. If a tea-spoonful is given by an empiric, its effects are fatal; but if the same quantity is administered by a learned doctor, and called grains, it is a useful medicine."

It is not necessary in this place to follow out the observations, of other writers on the Lobelia inflata, as I intend to introduce their observations in regard to its curative operations in the appendix to this article.

As regards its introduction into homœopathic practice, it was first noticed in my work on homœopathic practice, in which I detailed several cases of asthma, and other diseases, which were cured by this remedy in homœopathic dilution.

But the first publication of its pathogenesis was by Dr. Alphons Noack, of Leipsic, in his excellent treatise on the Lobelia inflata, in the fifteenth volume of the Hygea, (1841.) This exhibits very extensive research, and he has perhaps quoted every writer of any eminence who has mentioned this plant. To him I acknowledge myself indebted for a large portion of the references to previous writers, which are introduced into this paper.

The experiments of Noack were accompanied by contemporaneous thermometrical, barometrical and meteorological observations. Among the circumstances noticed in his experiments, on his own person, was the speedy decomposition of the urine passed on the first day of his trial of the lobelia. This had taken place by the next morning, when a rose red sediment was deposited on the sides of the vessel, in which was found a small brown urinary crystal, which under a microscope of two-hundred fold magnifying power, had the form and size of a large currant, and formed a glandular conglomerate. This observation is peculiarly interesting as confirmatory, on homœopathic principles, of my observations of its curative efficacy in cases when the urine possesses a copious lateritious sediment.

Noack's treatise has been translated and published, with slight abridgment, in the first number of the British Journal of Homœopathy.

The list of symptoms is generally accurately translated, but a few which occurred in cases of disease have been excluded. This is a liberty which I have carried to a greater extent, in excluding many of the symptoms which Noack has quoted from allœopathic physicians, because I find on reference to works in which the statements are made, that they do not appear substantiated by cases, and are some of them of a very doubtful character.

Besides the symptoms observed on himself, Noack gives the symptoms observed by the five following experimenters.

1. N. N. Kermes, a man aged 26 years, of venous lymphatic constitution, took 30 drops of the tincture in two ounces of water, at 9 o'clock in the morning, and 20 drops at 4 o'clock in the afternoon.

2. Medical student, Birkner, 23 years old, venous scrophulous constitution, took in the morning of the first day of experiment 4 drops of the tincture. In the morning of the next day 8 drops. In the morning of the third day 16 drops. A month afterwards he took 10 drops, and the next day 20 drops. A few days afterwards he took 40 drops.

3. Isidor Mortz, M. D., 29 years old; melancholic temperament; at the time of his experiment perfectly well, excepting a slight disposition to costiveness; took 10 drops three successive mornings, then 20 drops three

successive mornings; on the next day 30 drops; on the next day 10 drops in the morning and 10 drops in the afternoon; on the two following days 15 drops in the morning and 15 drops in the afternoon, and afterwards for several days with doses varying from 50 to 150 drops. He remarked that the small doses operated more upon the throat, the larger doses more on the stomach, and also that taking the tincture in water caused more extensive and continued operation.

4. Laura Kckh . . . . , 21 years of age, of a healthy family, graceful proportions, blooming countenance, with blue eyes, and brown hair, quiet, thoughtful and reserved disposition. In health at the time of the experiment. Took at night at bed-time 6 drops of the tincture, next morning and night the same dose; the following day none. The next day in the morning 9 drops, and the same at bed-time; the next day 9 drops in the morning 30 drops in the afternoon, and 40 drops at bed-time; the next day 50 drops at bed-time.

5. Dr. G. Otto Piper, of Dresden, commenced with a dose of 2 drops; the next day of 4 drops; the next day none; the next 6 drops; the next 7 drops; the next 8 drops the next 10 drops; the next day but one, 16 drops, and four days afterwards 20. He remarks that he could not prevail on himself to continue the trial farther, because the burning and prickling far exceeded in severity that of mezereum, ledum, polygonum and euphorbia, and the continued nauseous movement excited by the large doses really tormented him, and were a great hindrance to him in his indispensable occupations.

The names of those experimenters are marked with their initials, with the exception of Noack whose name, like those of other observers, is always printed in full after his own symptoms. The symptoms marked *Z——s*, were observed by a physician, who had taken the tincture in tea-spoonful doses every fifteen minutes, until nearly an ounce had been taken, without producing vomiting. The symptoms marked *N——n*, appear to have been inserted by the English translator of Noack's treatise.

HEAD.—Vertigo, with nausea. (*Williamson. Jeanes.*)

Vertigo, with pain in the head, and trembling agitation of the whole body. (*Williamson.*)

Dull feeling in the head after dinner, increased in the evening to violent pressive pain, with considerable heat of the face. (*B.*)

Pain in the head. (*Link.*)

5. Headache, with slight giddiness; occasionally transient shooting in the temples. (*K.*)

Dull feeling in the occiput. (*Geist.*)

Dull feeling in the occiput and forehead. (*Noack.*)

Pressive pain in the occiput, one while accompanied by heat, at another relieved by removing the covering from the head. (*B.*)

Pain in the occiput. (*Jeanes.*)

10. Dull heavy pain passing round the forehead, from one temple to the other, on a line immediately above the eye-brows. (*Jeanes.* In numerous cases, both of pathogenesis and cure; the latter often preceded by homœopathic aggravation, of several days continuance.)

Pains through the head in sudden shocks. (*Williamson.*)

Outward pressing in both temples, at the same time a dull pressing in the flesh just above the left elbow, and the hand feels as if paralyzed. (*Geist.*)

Pain in the parietal protuberance on the left side of the head. (*Jeanes.*)

Heaviness in the head, and uneasiness in the back. (*Eckh.*)

15. Chilliness of the left side of the head, with a feeling as if the hair would rise on end. (*Geist.*)

EYES.—Pain and soreness in the right eye. (*Williamson.*)

Pressing pain in the eye balls, most in the upper parts. (*Geist.*)

Severe and frequent itching in the angles of the eye lids. (*Jeanes.*)

Itching in the angles of the lids of the left eye. (*Geist.*)

Smarting of the inside of the eyelids. (*Geist.*)

EAR.—Aching in the left ear. (*Jeanes.*)

Shooting pain, extending into left ear from a painful spot in the throat, situated about an inch to the left of the larynx, and on a line with its lowest cartilage. (*Jeanes.*)

FACE.—Heat of the face. (*B.*)

Perspiration of the face, accompanying the nausea. (*M.*)

25. A peculiar drawing feeling extending from the right side of the mouth to the right eye. (*Geist.*)

A chilly feeling in the left cheek, extending to the ear. (*Geist.*)

Slight drawing feelings, at one time in the left, at another in the right side of the lower jaw. (*Geist.*)

TEETH.—Dull pressing pain in the left molar teeth and temple. (*Geist.*)

MOUTH.—Disagreeable taste in the mouth, somewhat similar to that of a solution of corrosive sublimate. (*Z——s*, 24 hours after taking.)

30. Pungent taste in the mouth. (*Williamson.*)

Flow of clammy saliva. (*Link.*)

Flow of saliva in the mouth. (*Noack.*)

Soreness of the throat. (*Jeanes, B.*)

Dryness of the mouth. (*Williamson.*)

THROAT.—35. Burning in the throat. (*Williamson. Noack. M. B.*)

Dryness of the fauces, frequent spitting. (*N——n.*)

Dryness of the throat. (*Williamson. B.*)

Tough mucus in the fauces, causing frequent hawking. (*M.*)

Prickling in the throat. (*Noack. P. M.*)

40. Burning prickling in the throat, increased secretion of viscid saliva, nausea and eructations. (*Noack.*)

Prickling in the throat, eructation and burning sensation rising up from the stomach. (*B.*)

Dryness and prickling in the throat, not diminished by drinking, after dinner. (*B.*)

Unpleasant sensation in the upper and back part of the pharynx, as from swallowing saliva during smoking. (*N——n.*)

Sensation as if the œsophagus contracted itself from below upwards. (*B.*)

45. Feeling of pressure, as from a foreign body in the whole course of the œsophagus, down which it proceeds with a vermicular motion, but most strongly felt in a spot just below the larynx and in the epigastrium. (*Noack.*)

Drawing pain in the right side of the throat, which extends upwards to the ear. (*Geist. Jeanes.*)

* Sensation of a lump in the pit of the throat. (*Jeanes.*)

STOMACH.—Loss of appetite. (*N——n. B.*)

Hiccough. (*Link.*)

50. Slight, frequent flatulent eructation, with flow of water in the mouth. (*Eckh. B. Noack. M.*)

Flatulent eructation, with sensation of acidity and heat of stomach. (*Geist. Jeanes.*)

Frequent violent hiccoughs, following each other quickly from twenty-four to thirty times, with abundant flow of saliva in the mouth. (*B. M.*)

Eructation of an acid fluid with burning sensation. (*Williamson.*)

Incessant violent nausea, with shivering and shaking of the upper part of the body.

55. An indescribable feeling about the stomach, compounded of nausea, pain, heat, oppression and excessive uneasiness, accompanying the affection of the respiratory organs. (*Z——s.*)

Nausea, great uneasiness and vomiting.

Nausea with great inclination to vomit.

Vomiting with cold perspiration of the face. (*M.*)

Extreme nausea, with profuse perspiration, copious vomiting, great prostration of strength, but good appetite shortly afterwards. (*Thomson.*)

60. Feeling of weakness of the stomach. (*Z——s, M. Jeanes.*)

* Sensation of excessive weakness at the præcordium extending upwards into the chest, and downwards as far as the umbilicus. (*Jeanes.*)

Feeling of pressure in the stomach, and extending to the back. (*Noack.*)

Feeling of weight in the stomach. (*Noack.*)

Sensation of oppression at the epigastrium, as if the stomach were too full; worse on pressure. (*Link.*)

65. Burning pain in the stomach towards the back, as if the part of the stomach nearest the spine were inflamed. (*N——n.*)

Violent painful constriction in the region of the cardia. (*M.*)

Warmth in the stomach. (*B.*)

Burning in the stomach. (*Williamson.*)

Heartburn and running of water in the mouth. (*B.*)

70. * Heartburn of long duration. (*Jeanes.*)

ABDOMEN.—Pain in the right hypochondrium. (*Jeanes.*)

Distension of the abdomen, with shortness of breath. (*K.*)

Flatulent rumbling in the abdomen, with pain. (*B.*)

Slight pain, sensation of motion in the abdomen, and escape of offensive flatus. (*Noack.*)

75. Pain in the abdomen, always worse after eating. (*Eckh.*)

Dull pain in the abdomen. (*Link.*)

Some pain in the lower part of the abdomen. (*Geist.*)

Sensation in the abdomen, as if diarrhœa was about to occur. (*Williamson.*)

Pappy stools. (*B. K.*)

80. Whitish, soft stools. (*Williamson.*)

ANUS.—Scraping sensation as from the passage of a rough hard body, during stool. (*Williamson.*)

Discharge of black blood, after stool. (*Williamson.*)

* Copious hæmorrhage from the hæmorrhoidal vessels. (*Jeanes.*)

URINE.—Desire to urinate and increased secretion of urine. (*Noack.*)

85. Increased secretion of urine. (*K. Noack.*)

Diminished secretion of urine. (*Noack.*)

Urine with a loose cloudy sediment. (*B.*)

Urine easily decomposed, and depositing a pink sediment, with a small brown crystal. (*Noack.*)

* Urine of a deep red colour, depositing a copious red sediment. (*Jeanes.*)

90. Sticking pain in the region of the right kidney. (*Geist.*)

Pain in the loins. (*Jeanes.*)

SEXUAL.—[Uterine hæmorrhage? *Gosewisch.*]

Pains in the sacrum. (*Eckh.*)

* Violent pain in the sacrum, with fever, etc., supervening suppression of the menses during their flow. (*Noack.*)

95. Aching pain in the urethra. (*Williamson.*)

Smarting of the prepuce. (*Williamson.*)

Troublesome feeling of weight in the genitals. (*P.*)

COUGH.—Sneezing, accompanying gaping and flatulent eructation. (*Geist.*)

Coughing. (*K. Geist.*)

100. Frequent, short, dry cough. (*Geist.*)

CHEST.—A general tightness of the chest, with short and somewhat laborious breathing. Discovered that he had a disposition involuntarily to keep his mouth open to breathe. (*Z——s.*)

Oppression of the chest. (*Link.*)

A tightness of the breast, with heat in the forehead. (*Geist.*)

Sensation of fulness in the chest, breathing somewhat short and superficial. Twenty-four respirations in a minute. (*B.*)

105. Oppression causing a deep breath to be taken. (*Noack.*)

Deep inspiration causes a feeling of comfort, from relieving the pressive pain in the epigastrium. (*Noack.*)

Oppression of breathing, acceleration of breathing,

with the feeling as if it were insufficient, and therefore required from time to time a deeper inspiration. (*B.*)

Abdominal respiration less than usual. (*B.*)

Inclination to sigh, deep inspiration. (*Geist.*)

110. Short inspiration, slow expiration. (*Geist.*)

Great difficulty of holding the breath. (*B.*)

A peculiar feeling, between tickling and smarting in the larynx, like irritation to cough, which, however, occurred but seldom, and then was accompanied by a feeling of oppression. (*Geist.*)

Slight tickling, on taking a deep breath, under the lower part of the sternum. (*B.*)

Sensation of a lump in the throat-pit, impeding respiration and deglutition. (*Williamson.*)

115. * Chronic dyspnœa, with the sensation of a lump in the pit of the throat, immediately above the sternum, impeding respiration and deglutition. (*Jeanes.*)

* Paroxymsal asthma. (*Cutler, Barton, Jeanes, and others.*)

Pains in the chest, increased by deep inspiration. (*B.*)

Pain in the breast. (*Geist.*)

Pains in the chest after walking after dinner. (*Eckh.*)

120. Burning feeling in the breast, passing upwards. (*Geist.*)

Slight deep-seated pain in the region of the heart. (*Geist.*)

Pain under the middle of the sternum. (*Geist. Link.*)

Burning pain in a small spot under the right breast, near the epigastrium; on a quick movement of the body, deep breathing, sneezing, and the feeling as if something had fallen out of its place, which went back again with great pain. The same pain in the epigastrium and left side. (*Eckh.*)

Violent boring pain through the back, under the right shoulder, extending from the painful place through the body, becoming more violent by motion. The painful place as if palsied. (*Eckh.*)

125. Pressing pain at the left side of the lower part of the sternum. (*Geist.*)

Feeling of drawing in the left breast, from the nipple to the axilla. (*Geist.*)

Pain about the third, fourth, and fifth dorsal vertebræ. (*Jeanes.*)

Rheumatic pains between the scapulæ. (*Geist.*)

Slight drawing pain between the scapulæ; previously slight muscular twitches over the ribs of the left side near the spine. (*Geist.*)

EXTREMITIES.—130. [Slight rheumatic feeling in the right shoulder-joint. (*Geist.*)]

Pain, only when touched, in the muscles of the right arm, in a space of the width of the hand, the pain in the shoulder gone. (*Geist.*)

Fine crawling stitches on the inside of the right deltoid muscle. (*Geist.*

Paralytic feeling in the left arm. (*Geist.*)

Pain in the right elbow-joint. (*Geist.*)

135. Severe rheumatic pain in the right elbow-joint. (*Williamson.*)

Pressing pain on the exterior, middle part of the thigh, and at the same time constrictive feeling in the head. (*Geist.*)

* Inflammatory rheumatism of the right knee, with swelling and extreme pain. (*Williamson.*)

Violent spasmodic pain in the left posterior iliac region, scarcely allowing touch or motion. (*P.*)

Violent tearing pain in the fibula, from below up to the knee-joint. (*P.*)

140. Pain in the left leg, whilst sitting. (*Geist.*)

A feeling about the knees of pain and stiffness, as from fatigue. (*Geist.*)

Weariness in the limbs. (*Eckh.*)

Cramp-like feelings in the left gastrocnemius. (*Geist.*)

Cramp in the calf of the leg, on awaking from a restless sleep. (*Eckh.*)

145. Cramp-like feeling in the hollow of the left foot. (*Geist.*)

Prickling sensation through the whole body, extending even to the fingers and toes. (*Cutler. Williamson.*)

Lobelia is felt in the fingers and toes. (*Thomsonians.*)

Frequent yawning and stretching. (*B.*)

GENERAL.—Shivering through the whole body. (*Eckh.*)

150. Feeling of weariness. (*B.*)

Uunusual weariness. (*P.*)

Heat, and inclination to perspiration, particularly in the face. (*B.*)

Chills down the back, with heat in the stomach. (*Jeanes.*)

* Intermittent fever.

155. Pulse more frequent, and weaker than usual, in the evening. (*B.*)

Pulse slower than usual. (*Noack.*)

Pulse of the usual frequency, but smaller and weaker. (*Jeanes.*)

Prostration of strength. (*Jeanes.*)

Restless sleep, with many dreams, also anxious dreams. (*Eckh.*)

160. Sad dreams. (*M.*)

Sleep disturbed at night by numerous dreams and frequent wakings. (*Link.*)

Sobbing like a child. (*Thomson.*)

APPENDIX.

The Lobelia inflata has been found both in large and in small doses a very valuable remedy in certain forms of asthmatic disease. Of its curative powers in these disorders, we have the testimony of Barton, Stewart, Randall, Bradstreet, Reece, Andrew, John Forbes,

Elliotston, Cutler, Bidault de Villiers, Behrend, Neumann, Sigmond, and others. That the relief afforded in some of the cases has been permanent, amounting to what may be properly termed cures, we also have satisfactory evidence. But its properties must be wonderful, if it can long sustain a reputation under this mode of application. Only adapted to relieve or to cure certain forms of asthma, but employed without discrimination for all, it must oftener be employed in cases where it is unsuitable, than in those which it suits. Whilst in some of the former cases no other inconvenience may be apparent than that arising from its medicinal operations, yet in others it may aggravate the existing symptoms, and add much to the sufferings and danger of the patients. This brings forward a mass of counter-testimony as to its applicability as a remedy, under the opprobrium of which it would decline into disuse.

That it has relieved, in doses of a few drops of the tincture, we have the testimony of Noack; but whether this mode of application has much to recommend it, time, observation and experience must determine.

That it has effected cures in the infinitesimal, minute doses of the homœopathist, I have the evidence of numerous cases in my own practice; that these cures would not have taken place had the remedy been administered in emetic doses, or in Noack's drop doses, I cannot assert. I can only be certain that they did take place after the administration of the minute doses, and according to my judgment in consequence of such administration. But it must be allowed, that if the minute dose answers only as well as the larger, it is much to be preferred, on the grounds of pleasantness and convenience.

Noack has arrived at the conclusion that its operation is peculiarly directed on the pneumogastric nerve, an opinion which is strongly supported both by its pathogenesis, and its curative effects.

There are other operations of Lobelia inflata than those on the lungs and stomach which are worthy of attention. Eberle succeeded readily in the reduction of an incarcerated hernia, after an enema of the infusion of this plant. This might depend upon mere relaxation, as from blood-letting, the tobacco enema, &c. &c. But an experience of my own has made me suspect that it possesses some properties which render it peculiarly suitable as a remedy in hernia. A patient labouring under all the symptoms of incarcerated hernia which remained in all their violence, after the apparent reduction of the hernia, (most probably from a constriction of the sac,) received, when in an almost hopeless condition, a minute dose of Lobelia inflata. In the course of two hours the bowels, which had not been moved for several days, became open, and the symptoms of incarceration speedily disappeared. This may have been a spontaneous change, such as has occurred in other cases of hernia, but it is certainly calculated to call attention to the investigation of the Lobelia inflata as a remedy for incarcerated hernia.

Doctor Gosewisch, of Wilmington, Delaware, remarks, in a letter to me: "Among the symptoms of lobelia which I have seen until now, I do not find any thing said about hæmorrhages. At first Dr. Edward Caspari told me he gave lobelia to an elderly lady, (who had not menstruated for four years,) for a pain in the right shoulder; it relieved the pain and brought on menstruation. I gave the same medicine to a lady in the last stage of consumption, who had not menstruated for six months; it palliated the cough and brought the menses, which continued for some days, though of course in small quantity; she died about three weeks afterwards. A lady over fifty years of age, who had long ceased to menstruate, had, after taking lobelia for a cough, bleeding at the nose. I have now under my care a boy who, after taking a Thomsonian emetic, had every evening, after an hour's sleep, a violent raving, with flushing of the face and palpitation of the heart. This has yielded rapidly to homœopathic treatment."

In some forms of gastric disorder the Lobelia inflata

has been found a valuable remedy. Noack gives the two following cases of cardialgia.

Cardialgia simplex. A young man had suffered for many years from attacks of pressing in the stomach, which extended itself upwards into the breast, causing a feeling of oppression and accompanied by nausea, flowing of water into the mouth and disposition to vomit, but no vomiting. The attacks occurred at no certain intervals, and sometimes continued for a long time. He had already tried a variety of remedies, among others the Carlsbad waters, which at first afforded a little relief but after a time ceased to do so. At a time when there was considerable fever, he took two drops of the saturated tincture of Lobelia inflata, once a day for five days in succession; many green diarrhœal stools occurred, but the pressing at the stomach gradually diminished and by the sixth day was entirely removed. Nineteen months afterwards the patient still remained free from the disease.

Cardialgia biliosa. A servant maid, aged twenty-six years, of bilious habit, had suffered for a long time from cramp of the stomach, which showed itself by a severe pressing feeling in the epigastrium, and which was excited by certain kinds of food, or mental emotion, especially in the evening, and continued into the night. In October, 1839, after fright and vexation during the menstrual period, which caused a suppression, she complained of alternating heat and cold, nausea, bitter taste, thirst, vomiting of bile, severe pressing in the epigastrium after eating, and also whilst fasting, exacerbating in the evening; oppression and a feeling of anxiety in the breast, and pain in the sacral region; her tongue had a yellow coating, and her pulse was small, weak and slow. A drop of the tincture of lobelia was given morning and evening, and by the second day produced marked effects. Severe pain in the forehead and frequent diarrhœal stools (seven in the day) took place, the vomiting ceased, the nausea diminished and the breast was no longer oppressed. A drop of the tincture on the third and fourth days removed the remaining bitter taste and the sacral pain. The patient was perfectly well by the fifth day.

To the above I add the following cases from my work on homœopathic practice, remarking that they have since been confirmed by many similar cures.

Case in a married lady æt. 38 ann. Accompanying chronic dyspnœa. Sensation of weakness and oppression at the epigastrium, and extending from thence into the chest. Burning in the stomach, and a sensation as if there was a burning lump in the pit of the throat, which appeared to impede swallowing and respiration. In swallowing, it seemed as if at this point something rose up to meet the food and obstruct its descent into the stomach. Frequent eructation of acid fluid with sensation of burning. Frequent vomiting of the food after meals, especially after eating warm food. She "had not known what it was to be without heart-burn for one hour for the last year." Her urine was high coloured, and deposited a copious red sediment. She had for a long time been subject to pain in the left lumbar region of the abdomen. Lobelia 4|6 effected a gradual but perfect removal of the whole train of her dyspeptic symptoms.

In numerous cases besides the above, I have succeeded in removing the dyspeptic symptoms by the employment of the same remedy. The chief indications for its use are—the sense of weakness and oppression at the epigastrium, and at the same time some oppression at the breast. But the nearer the approach of the symptoms has been to those of the above case, the less have I been disappointed in my expectations of a strikingly beneficial operation of the lobelia. There are, however, some cases where, although the symptoms of pectoral oppression are very trifling, yet this remedy operates satisfactorily. In a case of this kind, which I have but recently treated, and which occurred in a fat and robust man about 45 years of age, who complained chiefly of a copious hæmorrhoidal discharge and consequent debility, and a sensation of tightness in the epigastrium and some acidity of stomach. I at first gave him nux vom. without any apparent abatement of his disease, and subsequently some other remedies with the same want of success. At length he complained of some oppression at the breast, for which I administered lobelia 5|6. The following day he informed me that he felt new life and vigour, and that the pectoral, gastric and hæmorrhoidal disorders had all disappeared. Since that time, now about two weeks, he has remained free from them, and also from a feeling of want of power in the anus and rectum which was exceedingly uncomfortable to him while at stool, and to which he had been subject for many years.

In bleeding from the hæmorrhoidal vessels the Lobelia inflata has proved useful in the case just mentioned, and also in my own person.

The following cases show that as a remedy for some forms of intermittent fever it is deserving of attention.

Febris intermittens quotidiana. Attack at 10½ o'clock, A. M. In a man æt. 49 ann. Severe coldness, alternating with flashes of heat till 12 M., when the heat, which was moderate, became more constant, but alternating with slight chilliness, continuing till evening. Profuse sweat at night, slept during the sweat as usual. Thirst great from the first chill and during the whole of the hot stage, but worse in the chill. Respiration short, anxious, laborious and wheezing, with sensation of tightness of the chest. Sensation of oppression and weakness, principally at the epigastrium, but extending thence through the whole breast. Tickling in the pit of the throat, with frequent hacking cough. Severe headache, extending round the forehead from one temple to the other. Loss of appetite, both in the paroxysm and apyrexia. Tongue white, scaly, coated on the right side, but clean on the left. Great debility. Lobelia inflata 15|15, given at 3½ o'clock, P. M., during the paroxysm, produced considerable relief of the oppression of the respiratory organs, and the next day there was a very slight paroxysm, of short duration; the third day and afterwards no more.

Febris intermittens. Chill (shaking chill) with thirst, then heat with thirst and sweat. The thirst is sometimes observed before the chill and through the whole fever; often only before the chill, and not in it, and then again in the heat. The coldness is increased after drinking. The sweat begins with the heat, or after the heat has continued for some time.

The Lobelia inflata has by some been considered a valuable remedy in whooping cough. Noack remarks, that in some cases of whooping cough the lobelia appears to him to be even in the third stage (stadium adynamicum) of essential service.

The Lobelia inflata has not only been proposed as a remedy for croup, but it has also been extensively employed as such by the Thomsonians, and, from all that I have been able to learn, with a safety and success fully equal to that of the emetic treatment with the emetic substances in common use among other allœopathic physicians. But that the Lobelia inflata possesses properties which render it more adapted to the cure of croup than tartar emetic, ipecacuanha, squills, or senega, my observation has not led me to believe.

These medicines, by producing new and violent derangements, revolutionize the system, and thus frequently subdue the croup. They may sometimes, however, by their direct action upon the stomach, altering or removing the morbid condition, aid in a more direct, though still an indirect manner, in the cure of croup, where the irritation of the mucous membrane of the wind-pipe is sympathetic with gastric disorder.

Although the emetics above enumerated may often prove effectual remedies for the croup, yet we have only to compare the cases cured through the medium of their violent and stormy action, with those which are cured by hepar, spongia, phosphorus, and other remedies of similar powers, to enable us to appreciate the difference between cure by remedies of direct and indirect operation. The former, when given in sufficiently small doses, operate quietly and speedily, the local disease disappears as if by a charm, whilst the general health remains unimpaired by the remedy. The latter must be given in sufficiently large quantities to produce such great derangement of the actions as to overcome all minor derangements, involving them as the whirlwind involves the winds in its tempestuous vortex, and leaving, like the whirlwind, prostration and wreck behind.

So far as my observation extends, the Lobelia inflata is not to be considered a homœopathic remedy for croup: that is, a remedy possessing that power of directly modifying the condition of the parts most affected in croup, in such a manner as to effect a cure of this disease when given in small alterative doses. If there are any conditions of the system under which it exerts a decided influence of this character, further experience and knowledge of the remedy may show.

It will be proper to add, to what has already been said, some cases of cures effected by the use of the Lobelia inflata.

Asthma. Dr. M. Cutler narrates his own case as follows : " It has been my misfortune to be an asthmatic for about ten years. I have made trial of a great variety of the usual remedies with very little benefit. In several paroxysms I had found immediate relief, more frequently than from any thing else, from the skunk-cabbage, (*Dracontium fœtidum*, Lin., *Arum Americanum*, Catesby.) The last summer I had the severest attack I ever experienced. It commenced early in August, and continued about eight weeks. Dr. Drury, of Marblehead, also an asthmatic, had made use of the Indian tobacco, by the advice of a friend, in a severe paroxysm early in the spring. It gave him immediate relief, and he has been entirely free from the complaint from that time. I had a tincture made of the fresh plant, and took care to have the spirit fully saturated, which I think is important. In a paroxysm, which perhaps was as severe as I ever experienced, the difficulty of breathing extreme, and after it had continued for a considerable time, I took a table-spoonful. In three or four minutes my breathing was as free as it ever was, but I felt no nausea at the stomach. In ten minutes I took another spoonful which occasioned sickness. After ten minutes I took the third, which produced sensible effects upon the coats of the stomach, and a very little moderate puking, and a kind of prickly sensation through the whole system, even to the extremities of the fingers and toes. The urinary passage was perceptibly affected by producing a smarting sensation on passing urine, which was probably provoked by stimulus upon the bladder. But all these sensations very soon subsided, and vigour seemed to be restored to the constitution which I had not experienced for years. I have not since had a paroxysm, and only a few times some small symptoms of asthma. Besides the violent attacks, I had scarcely passed a night without more or less of it, and often so as not to be able to lie in bed. Since that time I have enjoyed as good health as, perhaps, before the first attack." He afterwards further remarks that, "in all instances of which I have had information, it has produced immediate relief, but the effects have been different in different kinds of asthma, some patients have been severely puked with only a tea-spoonful, but in all cases some nausea seems to be necessary. The asthma with which I have been afflicted, I conceive to be of that kind which Dr. Bree, in his practical inquiries on disordered respiration, &c., calls the first species, "a convulsive asthma from pulmonic irritation of effused serum." My constitution has been free, I believe, from any other disorder, than what has been occasioned by an affection of the lungs, anxiety of the præcordia, and straitness of the breast, and other symptoms produced by that affection."

Dr. William P. C. Barton states, that he administered it to a domestic in his family, "who was distressingly affected with spasmodic asthma. She is a female of narrow and depressed thorax, and for years past has been subject to this complaint. During one of the paroxysms I directed her to take a tea-spoonful of the brandy tincture every two hours. After taking the second spoonful, she was immediately relieved. In a subsequent attack, the experiment was repeated, increasing the dose to a tea-spoonful every hour, with the same effect; the patient declaring that she never found such immediate, and entire relief, from any of the numerous medicines she had previously taken for this complaint. She complained of dizziness, nausea, and some debility after taking the second spoonful."

Dr. Alphons Noack, of Leipzig, narrates the following case.

"*Asthma.* A lady in the climactric years, of bilious constitution, choleric temperament and great excitability, in a high degree hysterical, who had been married young, and since then been attacked from time to time by severe constrictive pains of the chest, uninterrupted hiccough, a jerking out of sounds which resembled a disagreeable laughter, and distortion of the muscles of the face. The paroxysms, when less severe, consisted only of loud sighing, moaning, with hurried expiration; the abdominal muscles worked strongly, the hands were firmly pressed upon the breast, the countenance presented the expression of a painful smile, and the pulse, with the skin at the ordinary temperature, was small, oppressed and slow. After some five minutes, longer and less noisy expiration, and long drawn sighs occurred, the patient became able to speak, opened her eyes, complained of great thirst, severe pain in the breast, epigastrium, hypochondria and loins, and of great debility. After short pauses, new attacks supervened on each other for many hours. The paroxysms were awaited in a lying posture, with the head drawn back. Strong mental emotion and frequent social dissipation, especially through the whole night, brought on these paroxysms, which mostly appeared in the early morning hours, and then did not repeat themselves for twenty-four hours. The habitual disorders of the patient consisted, moreover, in day sleepiness, nightly sleeplessness, twitching in the sleep, before going to sleep restlessness, heat in the hands and feet, which were at other times cold; shortness of breath from somewhat severe exertion of the body, pressing pain in the forehead, and frequent vomiting of water, with otherwise good digestion. In the earlier periods of her disease numerous medicines, from the so-called class of the volatile remedies, as musk, &c., also many mineral waters, were prescribed, but without success. I also had no cause to congratulate myself on my success with the many remedies I had employed, until I resolved to administer the lobelia. For a length of time I allowed her to take, evening and morning, a drop of the tincture on sugar, and during the attacks the same dose every quarter of an hour. The result was tolerably satisfactory, inasmuch as, at times, the disease only gave intimations of approach, without coming to an outbreak, and also when this happened they were both far less severe and of shorter duration; instead of the moaning presenting only sighing. But this modification was all that the lobelia could effect, the disorder not yet being removed."

I proceed now to mention one of the many cases of asthmatic disease in which lobelia has proved useful in my hands.

Case of a married lady æt. 38 ann. the mother of several children. She had suffered since her childhood from dyspnœa, increased by any active exertion, by going up or down stairs, by exposure to cold, and eating very warm food. Pain in the left lumbar region of the abdomen (also from childhood.) Within the last year, constant burning in the stomach and throat, with a sensation of dryness in the latter, as also of a lump in the pit of the throat which impeded respiration and deglutition. Weakness and oppression in the epigastrium with other symptoms of gastric derangement. Urine of a deep red, depositing a copious red sediment. Lobelia inflata, 4|6 was given in the evening, and by next morning the sensation of lump and burning in the throat, together with the dyspnœa, had greatly diminished, and in a few days entirely disappeared. The urine also became perfectly normal in appearance. She has continued well, without perceiving a trace of the asthmatic symptoms and pain in her left side, which she had experienced from childhood.

The symptoms which I have found most strongly to indicate the lobelia, are constant dyspnœa, which is increased by slight exertion, and aggravated so much by slight exposures to cold, as to form a kind of asthmatic paroxysm. A sensation of oppression and weakness at the epigastrium, extending upwards from thence into the breast, with or without pyrosis and cardialgia. A sensation of a lump or quantity of mucus, or of pressure, in the pit of the throat. A pain extending around the forehead from one temple to the other. Pain in the back about the lowest dorsal vertebra. Pain in the left side of the abdomen, immediately below the short ribs. High coloured urine depositing a copious red sediment.

Since the preceding remarks were written I have been induced by the pathogenesis of the Lobelia inflata, to employ it in the following severe case of a disease, which, though generally termed bilious colic, might much more properly be called

Gastralgia biliosa. A robust man of 35 years of age, who had an intermittent fever suppressed about a week before by the employment of the sulphate of quinia, in grain doses frequently repeated, was attacked during the night with uneasiness of the stomach, which continuing to increase, he took, about 10 o'clock in the forenoon, a large dose of anti-bilious pills. In the evening the pain became excessively violent. It occurred in frequent paroxysms of most excruciating pain, chiefly in the region of the stomach, accompanied with the feeling of a heavy load, great nausea and a disposition to vomit. By pushing his finger down his throat, he was enabled to produce vomiting, and succeeded in bringing up some thick yellow bile. About 10 o'clock, I was called to see him, I found him bathed in a cold sweat, with great prostration of strength and very feeble pulse, I gave him a drop of the first centesimal dilution of the tincture of the Lobelia inflata in a little sugar. It was succeeded by a paroxysm even more violent than any of the preceding. In his agony he made the same efforts to accomplish vomiting as before, but succeeded in bringing up but little. As the pain in the stomach began to abate, he complained of violent pain in the top of the right shoulder, and shortly afterwards of pain in the back, from about the first to the fourth dorsal vertebra. This pain lasted for some minutes. He then laid down and appeared to fall into a light sleep, during which the hands became warmer, the skin dryer, and the pulse stronger. In about half an hour he had another paroxysm, the pain which was not half so severe as it had been before, was felt lower in the abdomen, and was accompanied by rumbling of flatus. Soon after this I left him, feeling very confident that the disease was subdued. As he was very anxious about the pills not having operated, I allowed him, after he had rested a short time, an enema of molasses and water, which was followed by a couple of stools in the course of the night. The next day I found him sitting up, but quite weak, though entirely free from pain, of which he had but little after the second paroxysm, which followed the administration of the lobelia. In this case, the pathogenetic operation of the lobelia in the production of the pain in the shoulder and back, (which he had not felt previously to its employment,) led me to anticipate the result of its action, and all happened afterwards as I expected. The power of this remedy to produce those identical symptoms I knew, and when the patient complained of them, it was plain to me that the remedy was strongly operating upon the system, and that on this ground I must view the increased violence of the paroxysm as a homœopathic aggravation, which must be followed by cure. The improvement of the condition after this paroxysm, so different from that in which I found him, confirmed these views, which were still further corroborated by the mildness of the next paroxysm which also proved to be the last. Some persons will no doubt attribute the cure to the enema, which would aid in the operation of the purgative pills taken in the morning. But I object to this view of the case, that the cure was almost complete before the bowels were open; in fact, that the bowels were opened in consequence of the cure, instead of the cure being a consequence of such opening.

LOBELIA CARDINALIS.

BY SAMUEL R. DUBS, M. D.

The Scarlet Lobelia, or Cardinal flower. Die rothe Cardinals blume, Germ. La Cardinale, Fr.

Spec. Char. "Erect, simple, pubescent, leaves ovate-lanceolate-acuminate, erose-denticulate, raceme subsecund, many-flowered, the organs longer than the corolla." *Barton.*

This plant is said to have been employed as an anthelmintic, by the Cherokee Indians. Little or nothing, however, appears to be known of its value as a vermifuge, or of its other properties.

Took ten drops of the concentrated tincture, in about the third of a tumbler of water, at ten minutes past 10 o'clock, A. M. After the lapse of several minutes, it produced a burning sensation, with stinging in the tongue and fauces, which lasted till 12 o'clock at night.

In twenty minutes after taking, felt a sticking, like the pricking of needles in the sole of the left foot, shooting inwards. Passed away in a few minutes.

Same sensation, thirty minutes after taking, in the inner part of the right thigh, just above the knee. 11½ o'clock, A. M. Dryness of the nose with fulness, followed by sneezing.

12 o'clock, M. Severe stitch in the left side of the chest, which compelled me to press with the hand to moderate it, as it nearly took my breath; it continued about ten minutes.

12¼ o'clock, P. M. Same sticking pain in the left hypochondrium, which came on suddenly and so violently as to induce me to cry out. I placed the ends of my fingers over the spot, and the pain was at once moderated. Lasted about five minutes.

Bowels were opened about this time; stools at first thin, and then more consistent.

3 o'clock, P. M. Tongue raw, and sore, very red, especially at its tip, and a painful blister on that part.

Throat sore and dry, with disposition to swallow, as also to hawk up phlegm.

Headache dull and distressing, with fulness in the forehead and base of the occiput; the latter part was peculiarly painful. The pain increased by motion, or shaking the head.

5 o'clock, P. M. Severe pricking pain with itching in the heel of the left foot, so great as scarcely to be borne.

Headache increased, throbbing and weakness in the lower extremities, so much so, as to cause me to lie down. Hot sweat on the forehead, with throbbing in that part, and at the base of the occiput.

Stiffness of the nape of the neck. Dull pains in the upper maxillary bone of each side, with aching in the molar teeth.

Whilst lying down, great sleepiness, with difficulty of falling asleep. Constant dreaming with extreme lightness of the head. Starting in sleep, with jerkings of the hands.

7 o'clock, P. M. The soreness of the fauces is diminished, but the burning and pricking sensation remains the same. The soreness has extended lower down to the pharynx, and upper part of the œsophagus.

7½ o'clock, P. M. Unpleasant sticking pain in the epigastrium, which lasted five minutes.

9 o'clock. Very little pain in the forehead, but the pain is still throbbing, and almost insupportable in the occiput and nape of the neck.

Soreness in the eyes, with smarting and slight watering. Great repugnance to the light of a lamp.

10 o'clock, P. M. Oppression of the breathing, with dull and distressing pain in the lower part of the sternum, with the same feeling on each side forming a kind of circle. Relieved by beating lightly upon the part with the hand.

Dull heavy pain in the epigastrium, with sensation of a weight or load.

Dull distressing pain about three inches below, and a little to the left of the epigastrium.

Debility, and languor of the whole system, with weakness like from a sprain across the kidneys.

11½ o'clock, P. M. Slight shooting pain in the forehead, with an eruption of small vesicular pimples in the centre and upper part of this locality. They feel sore on passing the hand over them. The pain in the occiput is now very slight. Disposition to sing, which I was continually doing whilst walking up and down the parlour.

12 o'clock at night. Thirst for cold water, of which I drank half a pint. This very much relieved the pain and burning in the tongue and fauces. The pain and oppression at the breast were also alleviated.

Next day at 6 o'clock, A. M. Head feels light with dull pain in the forehead and occiput.

8 o'clock, A. M. Eyes burning and watery, with dread of light, and feel sore on closing them. Mouth and fauces dry, with a raw and distressed feeling extending down to the epigastrium. Some nausea, and still much distress at the epigastrium.

No appetite for breakfast.

Throughout the day great debility of the whole frame, but more especially of the lower extremities. They are so much fatigued by any exertion, that it is with difficulty that I can drag them along. My knees bend under me in walking.

August 13th. Sticking pains with sensation of a load at the epigastrium. Dryness and rawness, from the mouth to the epigastrium.

Appetite still very indifferent.

Oppression of the breathing through the day, with sticking pains on taking a long breath. Pricking pain in the left lung, coming on several times during the day, and lasting for several minutes each time.

Great weakness of the lower extremities.

Unpleasant taste in the mouth in the morning, and through the day.

Prickings like from needles in the calf of the left leg and the heel, worse in the latter part.

Most of the above symptoms continued, though with less intensity for two weeks, and it was at least three weeks before my stomach recovered its usual tone, and my usual good appetite returned.

PODOPHYLLUM PELTATUM.

BY W. WILLIAMSON, M. D.

Synon. Anapodophyllum canadense.

Aconitifolia humilis, flore albo unico campanulato fructu cynosbati.

Vulgo. May-apple, Hog-apple, Mandrake, Wild-lemon, Ducks-foot.

German. Schildblättriger Entenfuss, Entenfuss, Fluss-blatt.

Dutch. Eendenpoot.

Nat. Syst. Juss. Ranunculaceæ.

Nat. Ord. Linn. Rhœadeæ.

Nat. Fam. Podophylleæ.

Class. Polyandria.

Order. Monogynia.

Gen. Char.—*Calyx.* Perianth inferior, of three large, coloured, ovate, ascending leaves, caducous.

Corolla. Petals about nine, orbicular, concave, plated at the margin.

Stam. Filaments numerous, very short; anthers oblong, large, erect.

Pist. German superior, roundish; style none; stigma obtuse, sessile, plicate, crenate.

Peric. Berry globose, crowned with the permanent stigma, one-celled, many-seeded.

Recep. Unilateral, large and pulpy.

Spec. Char. Stem erect, one foot high, two-leaved, one-flowered; leaves peltate, palmate, lobate; lobe cuneate, incised. Blooms in May. Flowers white. Fruit mature in the latter end of August, lemon-coloured, of the size of a large plum and slightly maculated with brownish dots; the pulp to the taste at first is faintly nauseous, but agreeably sub-acid, and much esteemed by many persons. It is said the pigeons of Carolina are fattened by eating it.

Root perennial, creeping, from three to six feet in length, about twice the size of a goose quill, of a rich yellowish brown colour externally, and feeble yellowish white within. The main root is round and smooth, except that it is interrupted every three or four inches by knuckled joints, from which grow out numerous light coloured fibres. One of these joints which mark the successively annual attachments of the stem is added to the length of the root every year.

The root of the Podophyllum peltatum, according to the chemical analysis made by Dr. Staples, contains resin, gum or mucilage, soluble in cold water, amadin, colouring matter, extractive matter, ligneous fibre, and a minute quantity of an insipid substance soluble in sulphuric ether, from which it crystallizes in minute acicular crystals.

The leaves and root are the parts used in medicine. The leaves emit a strong narcotic odour, and have a nauseous taste. The root has a fresh nauseous smell and somewhat bitter taste. In popular phrase the leaves are said to be poisonous, the root medicinal, and the fruit edible. The fruit is aperient.

The preparation of Podophyllum peltatum, chiefly used in collecting the symptoms which follow, was composed of equal parts of the alcoholic tincture of the root and a tincture of the leaves, made by rubbing them up with alcohol, and immediately expressing the liquid from them.

This plant is emphatically a native, as it is indigenous to North America only, and is found growing luxuriously throughout the boundaries of the United States. It chiefly inhabits rich, loamy woodlands, but is frequently found growing in meadows, near small streams, and other low grounds.

The most conspicuous effect of Podophyllum peltatum, when taken in the dose of twenty or thirty grains of the powdered root, is purgation: a still larger dose will occasionally produce copious vomiting. By many practitioners it is considered one of the most safe and active cathartics, being slower in its operation, and less nauseating to irritable stomachs than jalap; it produces liquid discharges, without much griping or other unpleasant effects.

Dr. Snow, a graduate of the University of Pennsylvania, experimented on this article, and submitted the following result, in his inaugural thesis in 1819.

"A decoction was made, by putting two ounces of the leaves to one quart of water, and boiling and simmering it to eight ounces. At nine o'clock in the evening half of it was given to a full grown dog, and in thirty minutes the remainder. In ten minutes after the last dose, the pulsations of the heart were very weak, and from fifty to fifty-five in a minute; a copious salivation was produced; increased at twelve o'clock, but no narcotic effect; at ten o'clock and again at twelve o'clock he vomited, and the next morning he was found dead. The vomiting having been almost incessant from twelve o'clock until he died."

"One drachm of the leaves, in powder, produced restlessness for a short time in a dog, but afterwards he appeared to be as well as usual.

"Six drachms of the extract were made from two and a half ounces of the leaves, and then formed into pills of two grains.

"1st experiment. One pill was taken; pulse natural, seventy-six strokes in a minute; in one hour it had gradually diminished to sixty-five strokes in a minute, and continued so for about two hours.

"2d experiment. Two pills were taken; pulse seventy-four in a minute, full and strong; in one hour it had diminished to sixty-one, and in two hours afterwards it was still the same, weak and small.

"3d experiment. Three pills were taken; pulse seventy-six, full and strong; in one hour it diminished to sixty-four, and in two hours more it remained the same, small and feeble, accompanied with slight nausea."

"In a case of severe cough, accompanied with remittent fever, pulse small and tense; two grains of the leaves were given every three hours; on the second day, the pulse being still tense, four grains more were given, and on the third day there was a complete intermission, and a permanent cure effected.

In a case of pleurisy, after a small bleeding, pulse full; six grains of the leaves were given every two hours, and on the fourth day the patient was perfectly restored."

Being endued with the power of diminishing the frequency of the pulse, and the property of purging, the Podophyllum peltatum has been considered by allœopathists especially adapted to the treament of inflammatory diseases, which, in their opinion, require brisk purging; and by some it has been considered useful in intermittent fever, independently of its purgative quality.

The root also often operates as an anthelmintic, and as such has been used by the Cherokee and other southern Indians.

We have the concurrent testimony of a number of practitioners as to its efficacy in the treatment of mercurial rheumatism, colica pictonum, intermittent, remittent and congestive fevers, dropsy, hepatic congestions, scrofulous complaints, cough, hemoptysis, catarrhal and other pulmonary affections.

The relative position which the Podophyllum peltatum occupies among the natural families of plants, and the medicinal properties it is already known to possess, fully justifies the opinion that it is destined to become one of the most important of all the valuable medicinal plants indigenous to this country.

Antidote. Nux vom.

Compare with: Ars., Bry., Nux vom., Puls., Sep., Sulph.

Dose. The attenuations made use of in collecting the following symptoms, were the 1*st*, 3*d*, and 15*th*.

Much may be expected from Podophyllum peltatum in the following diseases, when indicated by the similarity of the symptoms:

Congestions of internal organs, especially of the liver and spleen.

Congestion of the head, with derangement of vision.

Periodical diseases.

Sympathetic affections.

Disease of one organ interrupting the functions of another.

Hypochondriasis.

Indigestion.

Headache, from disorder of the digestive organs.

Diarrhœa.

Dysentery.

Prolapsis ani.

Hemorrhoids.

Asthmatic complaints.

Colica pictonum.

Rheumatism.

Rheumatic affections from the abuse of mercury.

Remittent fever.

Intermittent fever.

Dropsies.

Verminous diseases.

Diseases with a *slow pulse.*

Pleurisy.

Cough.

Heartburn.

Waterbrash.

Cholera infantum.

Diseases of children during dentition.

GENERAL SYMPTOMS.—Sudden shocks of jerking pains. (*Williamson.*)

The symptoms generally but especially the abdominal symptoms, are aggravated in the morning and better in the evening. (*Williamson.*)

SKIN.— * Softness of the flesh, with debility in children. (*Williamson.*)

* Moistness of the skin, with preternatural warmth. (*Williamson.*)

* Sallowness of the skin in children. (*Williamson.*)

SLEEP.—Sleepiness in the day time, especially in the forenoon, with rumbling in the the bowels. (*Jeanes, Ward and Williamson.*)

5. Restlessness in the fore part of the night. (*Williamson, Jeanes.*)

Sleepiness early in the evening. (*Williamson.*)

Too heavy sleep at night. (*Williamson.*)

Distress after the first sleep in the evening. (*Williamson.*)

Rising up in bed during sleep, without waking. (*Williamson.*)

10. * Restless sleep of children, with whimpering at night. (*Williamson.*)

Moaning in sleep, with eye lids half closed. (*Williamson.*)

Drowsy and difficult to wake in the morning. (*Williamson.*)

Unrefreshed by sleep, on waking in the morning. (*Husmann, Jeanes, Ward and Williamson.*)

* A feeling of fatigue on waking in the morning. (*Jeanes, Williamson.*)

FEVER.—15. * Chilliness while moving about during fever, and in the act of lying down, with perspiration immediately afterwards. (*Williamson.*)

* Chilliness when first lying down in the evening, followed by fever and sleep, which is disturbed with talking, and imperfect wakings. (*Williamson.*)

* Fever attended with constipation. (*Williamson.*)

* Fever with incoherent talking. (*Williamson.*)

Intermittent fever, quotidian, *tertain* and quartan. (*Williamson.*)

20. * Chill in the morning at 7 o'clock, with pressing pains in both hypochondriæ, and dull aching pains in the knees and ankles, elbows and wrists. (*Williamson.*)

* Backache before the chill. (*Williamson.*)

* The shaking and a sensation of coldness continues for some time after the heat commences. (*Williamson.*)

* Some thirst during the chill, but more through the heat. (*Williamson.*)

* The patient is conscious during the chill, but cannot talk because he forgets the words he wishes to employ. (*Williamson.*)

25. * Delirium and loquacity during the hot stage, with forgetfulness afterwards of all that passed. (*Williamson.*)

* Violent pain in the head, with excessive thirst during the fever. (*Williamson.*)

* Sleep during the perspiration. (*Williamson.*)

* Loss of appetite in the apyrexia. (*Williamson.*)

HEAD.—Giddiness and dizziness, with the sensation of fulness over the eyes. (*Williamson*, *Jeanes.*)

30. Dulness and headache, with sleepiness in the morning. (*Jeanes*, *Williamson.*)

Momentary darts of pain in the forehead, obliging one to shut the eyes; attended with giddiness. (*Williamson.*)

Pain on the top of the head, when rising in the morning. (*Williamson.*)

Pressing pain in the temples in the forenoon, with drawing in the eyes, as if strabismus would follow. (*Williamson.*)

Stunning headache through the temples, relieved by pressure. (*Williamson.*)

35. Morning, headache with heat in the vertex. (*Williamson.*)

* Delirium and loquacity during fever, with excessive thirst. (*Williamson.*)

* Rolling of the head, during difficult dentition in children. (*Williamson.*)

* Perspiration of the head during sleep, with coldness of the flesh while teething. (*Williamson.*)

Sudden pain in the forehead, with soreness of the throat, in the evening. (*Williamson.*)

40. Vertigo while standing in the open air. (*Jeanes.*)

Vertigo with inclination to fall forwards. (*Williamson.*)

Headache alternating with diarrhœa. (*Williamson.*)

Heavy dull pain in the forehead, with soreness over the seat of the pain. (*Williamson.*)

* Morning headache with flushed face. (*Williamson, Jeanes.*)

45. Pain in the left frontal protuberance, aggravated in the afternoon. (*Williamson.*)

EYES.—Smarting of the eyes. (*Williamson.*)

Drawing sensation in the eyes, accompanying pain in the head. (*Williamson.*)

Heaviness of the eyes, with occasional pains on the top of the head. (*Williamson.*)

Pain in the eye balls, and in the temples, with heat, and throbbing of the temporal arteries. (*Williamson.*)

TEETH.—50. * Grinding of the teeth at night, especially with children during dentition. (*Williamson.*)

The teeth are covered with dried mucus, in the morning. (*Williamson.*)

MOUTH.—Copious salivation. (*Williamson.*)

* Offensive odour from the mouth. (*Williamson.*)

* Offensiveness of the breath at night, perceptible to the patient. (*Williamson.*)

55. The taste of fried liver in the mouth at night. (*Williamson.*)

Sourness of the mouth. (*Williamson.*)

Dryness of the mouth and tongue, on waking in the morning. (*Williamson.*)

* White fur on the tongue with foul taste. (*Williamson.*)

THROAT.—Soreness in the left side of the throat, especially painful when swallowing liquids, and worse in the morning. (*Williamson.*)

60. *Dryness of the throat.* (*Williamson.*)

Soreness of the throat extending to the ears. (*Williamson.*)

* Rattling of mucus in the throat. (*Williamson.*)

* Goitre. (*Williamson.*)

* Sore throat commencing on the right side, and then going to the left. (*Williamson.*)

APPETITE.—65. * Voraceous appetite. (*Williamson.*)

* Satiety from a small quantity of food, followed by nausea and vomiting. (*Williamson.*)

* Regurgitation of food. (*Williamson.*)

Indifference to food. (*Williamson.*)

Loss of appetite. (*Williamson.*)

70. * Putrid taste in the mouth. (*Williamson.*)

Desire for something sour. (*Williamson.*)

* Moderate thirst during fever. (*Williamson.*)

Thirst towards evening. (*Williamson.*)

* Diarrhœa immediately after eating or drinking (*Williamson.*)

STOMACH.—75. * Sourness of the stomach. (*Williamson.*)

* Acid eructations. (*Williamson.*)

Acidity in the afternoon with an unpleasant sickly sensation in the stomach. (*Williamson.*)

* Nausea and vomiting with fulness in the head. (*Williamson.*)

* Vomiting of food an hour after a meal, with craving appetite immediately afterwards. (*Williamson.*)

80. * Regurgitation of food. (*Williamson.*)

Extreme nausea, continuing for several hours. (*Williamson.*)

Vomiting of hot frothy mucus. (*Williamson.*)

* Vomiting of food with putrid taste and odour. (*Williamson.*)

* Heartburn. (*Williamson.*)

85. * Waterbrash. (*Williamson.*)

Heat in the stomach. (*Williamson.*)

* Belching of hot flatus which is very sour. (*Williamson.*)

Sensation of hollowness in the epigastrium. (*Williamson.*)

Throbbing in the epigastrium, followed by diarrhœa. (*Williamson.*)

90. * Stitches in the epigastrium from coughing. (*Williamson.*)

* Food turns sour soon after eating. (*Williamson.*)

* Gastric affection attended by depression of spirits. (*Williamson.*)

ABDOMEN.—Fulness in the right hypochondrium, with flatulence. (*Williamson, Jeanes.*)

Stitches in the right hypochondrium, worse whilst eating. (*Williamson.*)

95. Sensation of weight and dragging in the left hypochondrium, close under the ribs. (*Williamson.*)

* *Colic, with retraction of the abdominal muscles.* (*Williamson.*)

Pain in the transverse colon, at three o'clock in the morning, followed by diarrhœa. (*Williamson.*)

Rumbling of flatus in the ascending colon. (*Jeanes.*)

Pain in the ascending colon. (*Jeanes.*)

100. Pain in the bowels at day light in the morning, which is relieved by external warmth and by bending forwards whilst lying on the side, but is aggravated by lying on the back. (*Williamson.*)

The pain in the bowels at first is attended with coldness, which is followed by heat and warm perspiration. (*Williamson.*)

Sensation of heat in the bowels, accompanying the inclination to go to stool. (*Williamson.*)

Twisting pain in the right hypochondrium, with the sensation of heat in the part. (*Williamson.*)

* Chronic hepatitis, with costiveness. (*Williamson.*)

105. * Fulness, with pain and soreness in the right hypochondrium. (*Williamson.*)

Sensation of flatus in the left hypochondrium. (*Jeanes, Williamson.*)

Faintness, with the sensation of emptiness in the abdomen after stool. (*Williamson.*)

* Cramp-like pain in the bowels, with retraction of the abdominal muscles, occurring at ten o'clock in the evening, and again at five in the morning, and continuing until nine. (*Williamson.*)

* Sharp pain above the right groin, preventing motion, in the latter months of pregnancy. (*Williamson.*)

BOWELS.—110. * Constipation, with flatulency and headache. (*Williamson.*)

* Constipation accompanying remittent fever. (*Williamson.*)

* The fæces are *hard* and *dry*, and voided with difficulty. (*Williamson.*)

Diarrhœa early in the morning, which continues through the forenoon, followed by a natural stool in the evening. (*Williamson.*)

* Chronic diarrhœa, worse in the morning. (*Husmann.*)

115. * Extreme weakness and cutting pain in the intestines, after stool. (*Husmann.*)

Evacuations of green stools in the morning. (*Williamson.*)

From six to eight evacuations in a day. (*Williamson.*)

Diarrhœa immediately after eating or drinking. (*Williamson.*)

* Fæces yellow or dark green. (*Williamson.*)

120. * White slimy stools. (*Williamson.*)

* Cholera infantum. (*Williamson.*)

* Evacuations, consisting of a darkish yellow mucus which smells like carrion. (*Williamson.*)

* Frequent chalk-like stools, which are very offensive, with gagging and incessant thirst in children. (*Williamson.*)

* Copious evacuations, with blueness under the eyes. (*Williamson.*)

Painful diarrhœa, with screaming and grinding of the teeth, in children during dentition. (*Williamson.*)

125. Stools muco-gelatinous, small and unfrequent. with flatulence, and pain in the *region of the sacrum.* (*Jeanes.*)

* Hot, watery evacuations. (*Williamson.*)

* Frothy mucous stools. (*Williamson.*)

* Food passes the bowels in an undigested state. (*Williamson.*)

Evacuations in the morning, attended with strong urgings in the bowels, with heat and pain in the anus. (*Williamson.*)

130. Flashes of heat running up the back, after stool. (*Williamson.*)

Sensation at stool, as if the genital organs would fall out, in females. (*Williamson.*)

Too much bearing down at stool, as if from inactivity of the rectum. (*Williamson.*)

Secretion of mucus from the anus. (*Williamson.*)

Chronic diarrhœa, with prolapsus ani at every stool, in children. (*Jeanes, Williamson.*)

135. * *Prolapsus ani, with diarrhœa* of six years standing in an adult. (*Williamson.*)

* Prolapsus ani of long standing. (*Williamson.*)

* Descent of the rectum from a little exertion, immediately followed by stool, or a discharge of thick transparent mucus, sometimes of a yellow colour, and mixed with blood. (*Williamson.*)

* The prolapsus occurs most frequently in the morning. (*Williamson.*)

* Constant pain in the lumbar region, which is worse during evacuation, and particularly *after* stool. (*Williamson.*)

URINE.—140. * Enuresis. (*Williamson.*)

* Involuntary discharge of urine, during sleep. (*Williamson.*)

* Diminished secretion of urine. (*Williamson.*)

* Suppression of urine. (*Williamson.*)

Scanty urine, with frequent voidings. (*Williamson.*)

145. * Frequent nocturnal urination, during pregnancy. (*Williamson.*)

GENITALS.—Sticking pain above the pubes, and in the course of the spermatic cords. (*Williamson.*)

* Retarded menstruation. (*Williamson.*)

* Suppression of the menses in young females, with bearing down in hypogastric and sacral regions, with pain from motion, which is relieved by lying down. (*Williamson, Jeanes.*)

* Leucorrhœa; discharge of thick transparent mucus. (*Williamson.*)

150. * Leucorrhœa, attended with constipation, and bearing down in the genital organs. (*Williamson.*)

* *Prolapsus uteri.* (*Jeanes, Husmann, Williamson.*)

* Symptoms of prolapsus uteri, continuing for several weeks after parturition, with rumbling of flatus in the region of the ascending colon. (*Jeanes.*)

Symptoms of prolapsus uteri, with pain in the sacrum, flatulence unfrequent, muco-gelatinous stools. (*Jeanes,* 3 cases.)

* Pain in the regions of the ovaria, especially the right. (*Jeanes, Williamson.*)

155. * Numb aching pain in the region of the left ovarium, with heat running down the left thigh in the third month of pregnancy. (*Williamson.*)

* Ability to lie comfortably only on the stomach, in the earlier months of pregnancy. (*Williamson.*)

* Swelling of the labia during pregnancy. (*Williamson.*)

* After pains attended with heats and flatulency. (*Williamson.*)

After pains, with strong bearing down. (*Williamson.*)

LARYNX.—160. * Cough, accompanying remittent fever. (*Williamson.*)

* Dry cough. (*Williamson.*)

* Loose hacking cough. (*Williamson.*)

* Hooping cough, attended with costiveness and loss of appetite. (*Williamson,* 2 cases.)

CHEST.—164. Pains in the chest, increased by taking a deep inspiration. (*Williamson.*)

Snapping in the right lung, like breaking a thread, when taking a deep inspiration. (*Williamson.*)

Inclination to breathe deeply; sighing. (*Williamson.*)

Shortness of breath. (*Williamson.*)

Sensation in the chest, as if the heart were ascending to the throat. (*Williamson.*)

169. Sensation of suffocation, when first lying down at night. (*Williamson.*)

Palpitation of the heart, from exertion or mental emotion. (*Williamson.*)

* Palpitation of the heart, with a clucking sensation rising up to the throat, which obstructs respiration. (*Ward.*)

Sticking pain in the region of the heart. (*Williamson.*)

Palpitation of the heart, from physical exertion, in persons subject to rumbling in the ascending colon, heavy sleep, and a feeling of fatigue on awaking in the morning, followed by drowsiness in the forenoon. (*Jeanes*, numerous cases.)

TRUNK.—174. Pain in the small of the back when walking or standing, with the sensation of the back bending inwards. (*Williamson.*)

Pain in the lumbar region, with the sensation of coldness, worse at night, and from motion. (*Williamson.*)

Pain in the loins, increased by a misstep and walking over uneven ground. (*Williamson.*)

Pain between the shoulders with soreness, worse night and morning, and increased by motion. (*Williamson.*)

Pain under the right shoulder-blade. (*Williamson.*)

Stiffness of the nape, with soreness of the muscles of the neck and shoulders. (*Williamson.*)

180. Pain in the nape with soreness, increased by motion. (*Williamson.*)

Pain between the shoulders, in the morning. (*Jeanes.*)

19

UPPER EXTREMITIES.—* Rheumatism in the left forearm and fingers. (*Williamson.*)

Weakness of the wrists, with soreness to the touch. (*Williamson.*)

LOWER EXTREMITIES.—Pain and weakness in the left hip, like rheumatism from cold, increased by going up stairs. (*Williamson.*)

185. Pains in the thighs, legs and knees, worse from standing. (*Williamson.*)

Weakness of the joints, especially the knees. (*Williamson.*)

* Slight paralytic weakness of the whole left side, of one year's duration. (In a girl 18 years of age, *Jeanes.*)

Cracking in the knee-joints from motion. (*Williamson.*)

Heaviness and stiffness of the knees, as after a long walk. (*Williamson.*)

190. Stiffness on beginning to move. (*Williamson.*)

Aching of the limbs, worse at night. (*Williamson.*)

Pain in the left knee, leg, and foot. (*Williamson.*)

Sharp pain in the outer and upper portion of the left foot. (*Williamson.*)

Coldness of the feet. (*Williamson.*)

195. Perspiration of the feet, in the evening. (*Williamson.*)

SANGUINARIA CANADENSIS.

Indian Puccoon. Blood-root. Red-root.

Sanguinaria. *Sex. Syst.* Polyandria, Monogynia. *Nat. Ord.* Papaveraceæ.

Gen. Char. *Calyx* two-leaved. *Petals* eight. *Stigma* sessile, two-grooved. *Capsule* superior, oblong, one-celled, two-valved, apex attenuated. *Receptacles* two, filliform, marginal. *Nuttall.*

A spring plant, abundant in all hilly countries from Canada to Florida, wherever there is a rich soil and shade in summer, but avoiding the sea coast and the high mountainous regions. It blooms as early as April, and the elegance of its leaves and flowers and its graceful growth is so great, peculiar and indiscribably beautiful, that no delineation of it has yet appeared sufficiently graceful to those who know it. In appearance somewhat similar to the Hepatica, its leaves are delicate, and of a grey-green, like those of the Celandine, its flowers white and deciduous like those of the poppy, all scarcely higher than a hand. The root is perennial, of the length and thickness of a finger, knotty, fleshy and præmorse. Root, stem and leaves contain a yellowish-red juice, like as the Chelidonium a pure yellow, and the Papaver a white.

The leaves continue their growth after the time of flowering; and when the seeds ripen, have a more common appearance, nearly resembling the asarum. This is considered the best time to dig the root, which is the only part employed; the leaves, and especially the seeds, being considered poisonous. The first knowledge of its medicinal use is said to have been acquired from the Indians. It has also attracted the attention of some physicians, who slightly investigated its properties, while it was yet a source of honour for the physicians of this country to study the natural history of a land so rich in valuable medicinal plants; and before the day when surgery assuming the upper hand, the study of botany was contemned, its professors dismissed, and its gardens converted into coffee-houses, until science curtailed of its fair proportions, crippled and withered, revenged itself by presenting to the world practitioners of medicine, who knew little more than to cut, carve and burn.

The following synopsis, A, presents the most important remarks and observations of those physicians who have written on the sanguinaria, whose treatises have come to our knowledge. It is to be observed, that there is in most, if not all of their statements, a generalizing mode of expression, and an absence of attention to aught that is distinctive or characteristic in the operations of the medicine, so that in almost every instance the same remarks are applicable to many very different medicines, and in some instances the remarks are equally applicable to nearly every article in the Materia Medica. That the medical science which was satisfied with such loose investigations, and such still looser statements of them, should have been trampled under foot by surgical medicine, excites in us no astonishment and but little regret. Not that the investigations of sanguinaria have been peculiarly objectionable in this respect; on the contrary, they are accurate in comparison with those of many remedies much more frequently employed, and whose names are familiar as household words to the profession.

The second division marked B, presents the symptoms, both pathogenetic and curative.

The division marked C, contains cases and symptoms which have been cured with the sanguinaria, whilst the division D presents the pathogenetic symptoms as they appeared to some of the experimenters.

A.—*Observations of the Old School.*

1. Barton, Smith, Tully and Ives recommend the root, as an emetic.

2. Zollickhoffer mentions it as sudorific, emetic and purgative.

3. Smith and Allen compare it to digitalis; Thatcher considers it like to this; Tully says that it unites the properties of scilla, ammoniæ, senega, digitalis and guaiacum, without their dangerous operations.

4. Barton mentions it as a very powerful medicine, but as one which, by injudicious administration, may have dangerous consequences.

5. Rafinesque, (Medical Flora, 278) declares it to be one of the most valuable medicines of this country, acrid, narcotic, emetic, deobstruent, sudorific, expectorant, vermifuge, escharotic and also stimulating and tonic.

6. Schœpf says, that it is given in gonorrhœa, the bites of serpents, in jaundice and bilious diseases, which Rafinesque considers doubtful

7. Colden gave it in jaundice; Thatcher says that it is the chief remedy in Rawson's Bitters, a specific for jaundice.

8. McBride, says (see Bigelow,) "in torpor of the liver, attended with colic and yellowness of the skin, a disease common in this climate, (S. Carolina,) I use the puccoon with evident advantage. We use it also in jaundice, but in this disease I do not trust exclusively to it."

9. Dr. Ives, of New Haven, recommends it in influenza, in phthisis and in hooping cough. He also states that given in large doses, sufficient to produce full vomiting, it often removes the croup, if administered in the first stages. He recommends it also as a remedy of importance in many diseases of the liver.

10. Tully says that in diseases of the lungs it is tonic.

11. Smith says, that he found it of great use in the incipient stages of pulmonary consumption, and that acute rheumatism and jaundice, were benefited by it.

12. McBride found it useful in hydrothorax, given in doses of sixty drops, thrice a day, and increased until nausea followed each dose. In a week or two the good effect was evident, the pulse being rendered slow and regular, and the respiration much improved.

13. Rafinesque recommends it in asthma.

14. Dr. Ives gave it in influenza, &c. See 9.

15. Many, says Rafinesque, depend entirely upon it in croup. Dr. Ives says the same.

16. Dr. Allen considers it a substitute for digitalis in coughs and pneumonia.

17. Rafinesque states that in severe and protracted cynanche, pneumonia, hooping cough, phthisis, &c., when the the inflammatory symptoms are in part overcome, it operates as a tonic, expectorant, sudorific and sedative, bringing down the pulse from 112 to 80.

18. In typhoid pneumonia, "in plethoric constitutions, when respiration is very difficult, the cheeks and hands become livid, the pulse full, soft, vibrating and easily compressed,—the blood-root has done more to obviate the symptoms and remove the disease," than any remedy which he has used. Of the infusion of a scruple or half a drachm of the powdered root, in half a gill of hot water, he gave one or two tea-spoonfuls every half hour, until it excited vomiting, or relieved the symptoms. *Dr. Ives.*

19. "It promises to be a useful medicine, particularly on the foundation of its emetic and expectorant effects, in cases of cynanche maligna, or ulcerous sore-throat, in cynanche trachealis, or hives, and other similar affections. Its properties seem to be considerably allied to those of seneca snake root, so beneficially employed in the same cases." *Barton.*

20. The decoction has been employed with advantage in sore-throat, also in that form termed by Darwin, peripneumonia trachealis. *Barton.*

21. In ulcerated sore throat, in dysentery, and in amennorrhœa. *Rafinesque.*

22. It is given in inflammatory rheumatism; it cures acute rheumatism, complicated with gout. *Rafinesque.*

23. Barton states that the tincture of the root used as bitters, increases the appetite and strengthens the stomach, and thus prevents fevers from marsh miasm.

24. Rafinesque says that in the South it is a common preventive remedy of intermittent and putrid fevers.

25. Schœpf says, that the plant is given to horses to make them sweat, and also when shedding the hair.

26. According to Schœpf, the juice is used to eat away warts.

27. Dr. Downey has employed it, with success, in old indolent ulcers, especially in ill conditioned ulcers, with callous borders and ichorous discharge.

28. According to Rafinesque, when externally applied to ulcers, and in diseases of the skin, it changes the actions, and favours secretion.

29. Applied to fungous flesh it proves escharotic, and several polypi of the soft kind were cured by it. *Smith.*

30. Barton says that he has "heard of the application of the powdered root to a fungous tumour within the nostril, with the effect of producing detumescence, and bringing away, frequently, small pieces of the fungus, which in the first instance impeded the progress of the air through the nostril, and was supposed to be a polypus.

31. Dr. Benj. Becker mentioned to me, that a polypus of the nose ceased to grow, from the time that the powder of the root was snuffed.

32. According to Rafinesque and others, it is a popular remedy for nasal polypus, fleshy excrescences, and spongy swellings.

33. "The sanguinaria has a faint narcotic odour, and a bitterish, very acrid taste, the pungency of which remains long in the mouth and fauces." *U. S. D.*

34. Rafinesque describes the taste as acrid and bitter in the mouth, and burning in the throat.

35. Barton says that "the tincture is intensely bitter, approaching in its permanent impression to acerb." Bigelow says that the tincture "possesses all the bitterness, but less of the nauseating quality than the infusion."

36. According to Barton, and others, "the powder creates great irritation of the fauces." Dr. Smith says of the powder, that when "snuffed up the nostrils, it proved sternutatory, and left a sensation of heat for some time."

37. Downey (Essay on Sanguinaria, Baltimore, 1803,) says, that twenty grains of the fresh root, or eight grains of the extract in alcohol or water, cause nausea and vomiting, a feeling of warmth or heat in the stomach, quickened pulse, and, in many experiments, slight headache. In all cases the acrimony of the medicine made a long enduring impression on the fauces, and in many cases moved the bowels.

38. Bird, (Dissertation on Sanguinaria, New York, 1822,) speaks of it as one of the best acrid narcotic remedies.

Ten to twenty grains operated as an emetic; larger doses caused suppression ofthe pulse, fainting, dimnness of vision, and very great prostration of strength.

39. Dr. Smith states that "he found the powder to operate violently as an emetic, producing great prostration of strength during its operation, which continued for some time."

40. Barton says, that "fifteen or twenty grains of the pulverized root produce powerful emesis; but the medicine must be given in the form of pills, as the powder creates great irritation of the fauces."

41. Dr. Dexter says, that "it proved efficacious as a stimulant, and diaphoretic in doses of one grain of the powdered root, or ten drops of the saturated tincture."

42. Rafinesque says, that in doses of from two to four grains, it causes nausea and vomiting, and quickened circulation; in doses smaller than a grain, that it

acts as a tonic, and diminishes the frequency of thé pulse like digitalis.

43. Rafinesque cautions against its use during pregnancy, as it acts very powerfully on the uterus, and causes abortion, and recommends its employment in amennorhœa.

44. Barton says, that the root "when exhibited as an emetic, has been found to dislodge worms from the stomach."

45. According to Barton and Downey, the leaves and the seeds are evidently deleterious. The latter produce effects similar to those brought on by the seeds of stramonium, exhibiting a very considerable influence over the pulse, and a stupifying narcotic quality.

46. The seeds act upon the brain, causing torpor, langour, dilatation of the pupils, and dimnness of vision.

47. The seeds are powerfully narcotic, like stramonium, cause fever, delirium, and dilatation of the pupils, yet have been used as a diuretic. *Rafinesque.*

48. According to Wibmer, says Richard, (Med. Bot. 1070,) the sanguinaria causes palpitation of the heart, nausea, weakness, fainting, diminished power of sight, and at times vomiting and purging.

49. The root is bitter and acrid to the taste, leaving a durable sense of acrimony in the fauces.

50. Employed in as large doses as can be taken without disquieting the stomach, and repeated regularly and at short intervals, it occasions increased secretions from the digestive viscera and a universal change of action or condition in the whole absorbent and secernent systems. (*Tully.*)

51. It resolves atonic, acute, sub-acute and chronic inflammations of the thoracic and abdominal viscera. (*Tully.*)

52. Also arthritic inflammations of the muscles and joints. (*Tully.*)

53. It frequently excites the appetite, and promotes digestion. (*Tully.*)

54. It occasions a gradual and moderate increase of the force and fulness of the pulse. (*Tully*.

55. It is sometimes expectorant. (*Tully*.)

56. It is sometimes emmenagogue. (*Tully*.)

57. It has been known to produce uterine hæmorrhage. (*Tully*.)

58. In large doses it strongly nauseates. (*Tully*.)

59. It powerfully abates irritative hardness, and frequency of the pulse.

60. Also irritative heat and dryness of the skin.

61. It usually occasions a quickly diffused and transient heat, but at the same time a very peculiar nervous thrill, which is often extended to the minutest extremities.

62. In large or full emetic doses, it speedily excites the action of vomiting, but without the production of much nausea or any perceptible, or at least material diminution of the energies of the system.

63. In inordinate doses, "it sometimes occasions vomiting, but more especially burning at the stomach, faintness, vertigo, diminished vision and general insensibility, coldness, extreme reduction of the force and frequency of the pulse, together with great irregularity of action and palpitation of heart, great prostration of muscular strength, and sometimes (though in all probability rarely,) a convulsive rigidity of the limbs." (*Tully*.)

B.—*Symptoms occurring in trials of Sanguinaria upon the healthy.*

Extreme moroseness. (*Bute.*) Anxiety before the vomiting, (*Bute*, 130) and before the delirium, which is caused by the seed. (A, 47.)

Vertigo, &c.

Vertigo, with singing in the ears, flatulent eructation and then tickling in the throat which excites cough. (Immediately after taking it.)

Frequent vertigo and diminished vision before vomiting, (A, 40,) and after large doses. (A, 63.)

Vertigo with nausea, (A, 48,) long continuing with debility, (*Bute.* 138,) with head-ache. (24.)

5. * Vertigo on quickly turning the head, and looking upward. (C, 1.)

Confused and dull feeling in the head, which became better after eructation. (Soon after taking it.)

Determination of blood to the head, with whizzing in the ears and a transitory feeling of heat; then a sensation as if vomiting was about to take place, but instead of this there succeeded slight cutting drawings in the abdomen, and then a stool.

Heaviness in the head.

Dull pain in the head.

Pains in the head.

10. Slight headache from large doses. (A, 37.)

Pressing drawing in the forehead.

Pain in the forehead. (After five days. *Neidhard.*)

Pain of a short duration in the right side of the forehead, like a pressing, only whilst standing still, better whilst walking. At the same time a pain deep in the left ear. (*Husmann.* D, 22.)

Headache as if the forehead would split, with chill and with burning in the stomach.

A pain occurs suddenly in the interior angle of the right eye, and from thence to the forehead.

Headache on waking, in the forehead, on the right side, extends into the ear, at the same time toothache. (*Husmann.*)

About 5 o'clock in the evening a severe quick darting pain in the forehead and temple on the right side, which endured for about five minutes. This pain reappeared in the evening about 7 o'clock. About 11 o'clock at night a sudden pain through the forehead like an electric stroke of short duration.

A slowly shooting pain in the forehead. (*Jeanes.* D, 4.)

Periodic stitches in the left temple.

Pain in the top of the head.

Pain in all the upper part of the head.

In the afternoon, pain, like fulness, in the fore part of the head. (*Husmann*, D, 25.)

Pressing in the upper part of the head, in the region of the anterior fontanelle, disappears whilst walking. (*Husmann*, D, 26.)

Boring pain above, in the fore part of the head. (*Husmann*, D, 36.)

Severe pain above, on all the left side of the head, especially in the eye; at the same time similar pain in the left foot. (*K*, §.)

Nausea, disposion to vomit without being able to do so; then headache with rheumatic pains and stiffness in the limbs and neck.

20. Beating headache and bitter vomiting.

Headache in the evening, with tickling in the throat. (*Bute*. 191.)

Headache, with chill.

Headache, with nausea and chill, then flying heat from the head to the stomach.

Headache, with vertigo and pain in the ear. (*K*. §.)

25. Headache, whilst lying down.

Beating headache, worse by stooping.

Headache, worse by stooping and motion.

The beating headache is worse by every motion.

The headache occurs paroxysmally.

30. Pain in the head, of six hours duration.

* Pains in the head, in spots, soreness, especially in the temples. (C. 3.)

* Pains in the head, in rays drawing upward from the neck. (C. 6.)

* Severe pains in the head, with nausea and vomiting, frequently with bilious vomiting, in attacks with hebdomadal or longer intervals, from very different inducements, commonly beginning in the morning, increasing in violence through the day, only diminished by lying quiet, and when possible by sleep. North American sick-headache. (*Helffrich*, *Hering*.)

Feeling as if the head is drawn forward.

35. Soreness of the scalp, on being touched.

Feeling of looseness of the scalp on the right side.

Sensation of looseness and drawing in one side of the scalp, on raising the eyes.

Distension of the veins on the head.

* Distension of the veins in the temples, perceptible on touching. (C, 2.)

40. Feeling of fulness in the face.

Distension of the veins of the face, with excessive redness, and a feeling of stiffness.

Severe burning, heat and redness of the face.

Redness of the face.

* A red cheek, with burning in the ears. (C, 10.)

* Redness of the cheeks, with cough. (C, 13, 14.)

Paleness of the face, with disposition to vomit. (*Bute.* 124.)

* Cheeks and hands livid, in typhous pneumonia. (A, 18.)

Twitching of the cheeks, towards the eyes.

EYES.—50. Pain in the right eye.

Pressing pain in the left eye. (*K.* §.)

Stitch in the upper eyelid. (*K.* §.)

Watering and burning of the right eye, which is painful on being touched, then coryza. (B, 184.)

Feeling as if the eyes were affected by sour smoke. Afternoons about 2 o'clock. (*Husmann.* D, 31.)

In the afternoon dimness of the eyes, and a feeling as if hairs were in them.

55. Very great glimmering before the eyes. (*K.*)

Diminished power of vision. (A, 63.)

Dilatation of the pupils, by the seeds. (A, 46, 47.)

EARS.—Beating under the ears, at irregular intervals, frequently only a couple of strokes.

* Burning of the ears, with redness of the cheeks. (C, 10.)

60. Pains in the ears, with headache. (*Bute.* 24.)

Singing in the ears with vertigo. (*Bute.* 1.)

Humming in the ears, with determination of blood. (*Bute.*)

Slow stitches in the left ear. (*Jeanes.*)

Pain in the left ear, during the pain in the forehead. (C, D, 23.)

Beating humming (*wuwwern*) in the left ear.

In the neighbourhood of a smithy he feels every hammer stroke painfully, in the right ear.

A crackling in the right ear, when he draws his fingers lightly over his right cheek; on the left side this is not the case. (*Hering*. D, 30. The 3d day.)

NOSE.—65. Heat in the nose. (A, 36.)

* Nasal polypus. (A, 29, 32.)

* Loss of smell. (*Bute*. 93.)

Smell in the nose like roasted onions.

Dislike to the smell of syrup.

JAWS.—70. Stiffness in the jaws.

Pain in the upper teeth.

Pain in a hollow tooth, especially when touched by the food.

Tooth ache, from picking the teeth.

Pain in one or more of the incisor teeth, and in a carious molar tooth. (*Jeanes*. D, 11.)

Shooting and thrilling pain in a carious molar of the upper jaw, which passes away gradually in that form of pain which is often termed a grumbling toothache. (*Jeanes*. D, 12.)

On awaking, tooth-ache in an upper carious tooth, on the right side, at the same time headache in the same side. The toothache is made worse by cold water, (also by drinking hot things) and better by drinking warm drink. (*Husmann*. D, 15.)

Pain in a carious molar after cold drinking, two mornings in succession. (*Husmann*. D, 24.)

Looseness of the teeth.

75. Salivation and looseness of the teeth; he supposes himself able to take them all out. (Verbally through *Dr. B. Becker*.)

Spitting with nausea. (*Bute*, 113, 114, 115, 80.)

Feeling of dryness of the lips. (In three experimenters.)

THROAT.—Feeling of dryness in the throat, not diminished by drinking.

Heat in the throat, alleviated by the inspiration of cool air. Evenings, 6 to 7 o'clock. (*Husmann.* D, 35.)

A long continuing impression in the fauces. (A, 33, 35, 36, 40, 49.)

A transitory, but marked sensation in the fauces, as if he had swallowed something acrimonious. (*Jeanes.* D, 8.)

80. Burning in the fauces, after eating sweet things (*Bute*, 94.)

Burning in the œsophagus.

A feeling in the throat, as if it were swollen up; and would suffocate him, with pain in the throat on swallowing, and with aphonia. (After 3 hours, duration one hour.)

In the evening a pain with a feeling of swelling in the throat, worse on the right side, and most perceptible on swallowing.

Feeling of swelling in the throat on swallowing.

85. * Angina, in several cases, particularly a species of pharyngitis. (C, 4, A, 17, 19, 20.)

* Ulcerated sore throat. (A, 21.)

MOUTH.—A prickling sensation on the tongue, and roof of the mouth, as after chewing mezereum, but slighter. (*Jeanes.* D, 20.)

Crawling on the point of the tongue, after which an acerb feeling extends itself over the whole tongue, in the morning on awaking. (*Husmann.* D, 13.)

Prickling on the point of the tongue. (*Husmann.* D, 17.)

Tongue as if burned. (K.)

A feeling of dryness and rawness as after acrid things, begins on the right side of the tongue and spreads over the whole tongue, mornings on awaking. (*Husmann.* D, 18.)

* Tongue sore, pains like a bile. (C. 7.)

Stitches on the left side of the tongue. (*Husmann.* The third day. D, 34.)

90. White coated tongue with loss of appetite.
Loss of appetite with uncertain cravings. (*Bute.* 99.)
* Increases the appetite. (A, 23, 53.)
Loss of smell and taste.
A piece of sugar cake tastes bitter, followed by burning in the fauces.
95. Fatty taste in the mouth. (K.)
Slimy taste in the mouth.
Disinclination for butter, which leaves a disagreeable after-taste.
Dislike to the odour of syrup. (*Bute*, 69.)
Craving for he knows not what, with loss of appetite.
100. Craving for piquant food.
STOMACH.—Pressing in the stomach.
Soreness in the epigastrium aggravated by eating. (*Neidhard.*)
Feeling of warmth and heat in the stomach. (A, 37.)
Burning in the stomach, from large doses. (A, 63.)
Burning in the stomach, with headache. *Bute*, 12.)
Jerking in the region of the stomach, as if from something alive.
105. Great weakness of digestion.
Loss of appetite. (*Neidhard.*)
* Strengthens the stomach. (A, 23, 40, 50.)
Excites the appetite and aids digestion. (A, 53.)
Soon after eating, a feeling of emptiness in the stomach.
* Inflammation of the stomach. (A, 51.)
NAUSEA.—Nausea. (*Bute.* A, 12, 37.)
Severe nausea from large doses. (A, 58.)
Nausea as if vomiting would succeed. (From smelling. *Jeanes.*)
Nausea after eating.
110. Nausea which is not diminished by vomiting.
Loss of appetite and periodic nausea.
Nausea by stooping.
Nausea with much spitting.
Extreme nausea with great salivation.
115. Nausea with flow of saliva and constant spitting.
Long continued nausea with chill.

Nausea without vomiting, then headache. (*Bute*, 19.)

Nausea with the headache, with chill and heat. (*Bute*, 23.)

Nausea before the nettle-rash. (C, 23.)

120. Heartburn and nausea. (A, 40.)

Regurgitation and disposition to vomit. (*Bute*, 27.)

Flatulent eructation. (*Bute*, 1.)

Spasmodic eructation of flatus.

Hiccough, whilst smoking tobacco. (*Husmann*. D, 32.)

Frequent flatulent eructation of unpleasant odour, with disposition to vomit, and paleness of the face.

125. After the eructation of flatus, the dulness of the head becomes better. (*Bute*, 6.)

VOMITING.—Vomiting. (A, 1, 2, 5, 37, 38, 39, 40, 42, 48.)

Many unpleasant feelings previous to the vomiting. (A, 40.)

130. Before vomiting, great anxiety.

Before vomiting, slight pressure to stool. (*Bute*, 154.)

Vomiting of bitter water.

Bitter vomiting, with the headache. (*Bute*. 20.)

Vomiting, with craving to eat, in order to quiet the nausea.

135. Vomiting worms. (A, 44.)

Vomiting and diarrhœa.

Whilst vomiting, and afterwards, great weakness. (A, 39.)

Causes vomiting, without nausea or perceptible weakness. (A, 62.

ABDOMEN.—Severe and continual pain in the hypochondria; vertigo and debility.

* Pain in the left hypochondrium, worse by coughing, better by pressure, and lying on the left side. (C, 15.)

140. Diseases of the liver. (A, 19.)

Torpor and atony of the liver. (A, 8, 66.)

Inflammation of the abdominal viscera. (A, 51.)

Hot streamings from the breast towards the liver (*Husmann*. D, 37.)

Beating in the abdomen.

Cramp in the abdomen, which passes from one place to another.

* Sensation as if hot water poured itself from the breast into the abdomen, followed by diarrhœa. (C. 16.)

* Flatulent distension of the abdomen in the evenings, with the escape of flatus from the vagina. (C, 16.)

145. Discharges of flatus upwards and downward, by raising himself up on account of the cough, which then ceases. (*Bute.* 192.)

* Indurations in the abdomen.

Bellyache.

Paroxysmal pain in the abdomen.

Slight cutting drawings in the abdomen.

* Colic, with torpor of the liver. (A, 8.)

150. In the night, digging pain in the abdomen, with pain in the sacrum.

An hour after taking it, severe cutting pain in the bowels, followed by a single watery stool.

In the morning, colicy pain in the upper part of the abdomen, and then a diarrhœal stool.

Pressure to stool, without evacuation, with the sensation of a mass in the lower part of the rectum; this sensation recurred frequently during the day, without stool.

Inoperative pressure to stool, then vomiting.

Feeling of pressure to stool. (*Jeanes.* D, 1.)

155. In the afternoon frequent pressure to stool, but only discharges of flatus.

Urging to stool, with great discharge of flatus.

Frequent discharges of very offensive flatus; in the evening a hard stool.

Flatulent discharge, followed by a small stool, with relief of the sensation of pressure to stool. (*Jeanes.* After two hours. D, 9.)

Diarrhœal stools, with great flatulence.

Purges. (A, 25, 37, 48.)

160. After cutting pains, stool. (*Bute.* 37.) After

severe pains, stool like water. (151.) After colic. (152.)

In the evening diarrhœa, with disappearance of the coryza. (*Bute.* 184.)

* With the diarrhœa, termination of the coryza and catarrh. (C, 11.)

* Diarrhœa terminated the attack of pains in the breast. (C. 16.)

* Dysentery. (A. 21.)

165. The food passes away undigested in the stool.

Frequent natural stools, five times in the day.

Two small, but not fluid stools. (The 1st day. *Husmann.* D, 20.)

The first days the stools more laxative and frequent, afterwards rather costive. (*Husmann.* D, 45.)

* Hæmorrhoids. (C, 5.)

A twisting pain on the left side above the groin, equi-distant from the symphysis pubis, and the crest of the ilium; worse whilst sitting, standing or bending towards the right side, increased by pressure; better whilst walking erect. In the afternoon of the 8th day. Afterwards this pain passed towards the hip, around and upward, till it reached posteriorly on the short ribs, and remained peculiarly sensible by bending to the right. (*Husmann.* D, 44.)

URINE.—Frequent urination, also at night.

In the night frequent urination, the discharges large, of urine as clear as water.

170. The seeds are diuretic. (A, 47.)

* Frequent and copious nocturnal urination. (C. 15.)

Seminal emissions during sleep, two nights in succession, after which he feels very well. (From the 6th to the 8th day. *Husmann.* D, 40.)

* Gonorrhœa.

FEMALE.—Abdominal pains, as if the menses would appear.

The whole night abdominal pain, like the menstrual.

175. It at times aids menstruation. (A, 56.)

The menses appear a week too early, with a discharge of black blood.

Abortion, on account of too strong operation on the uterus. (A, 43.)

Causes uterine hæmorrhage. (A, 57.)

* Amennorrhœa. (A, 21.)

* Escape of flatus from the vagina, with dilatation of the os uteri. (C, 6.)

* Climacteric disorders. Compare mammæ and mamillæ.

The menses appear at the proper time, but still much more freely than at other times, with less pain and weakness in the sacrum, but with pain in the right side of the head and forehead, and a feeling as if the eyes would be pressed out of the head, worse on the right side. (The 7th day. *Husmann.* D, 17.)

CORYZA.—180. Much sneezing.

Fluid coryza, with frequent sneezing.

Severe fluid coryza in the right nostril.

Watery, acrid coryza, which renders the nose sore.

Copious watering of the right eye; the eye painful, especially on being touched; and soon afterwards there occurred a copious watery discharge from the right nostril; in the evening two diarrhœal stools, and then all the symptoms disappeared. (Five hours after taking it.)

185. Fluid coryza, alternating with stoppage of the nose.

Aphonia, with swelling in the throat. (*Bute.* 82.)

Tickling irritation to cough. (*Bute.* 1.)

* Influenza. (A, 14.)

* Coryza, rawness in the throat, pain in the breast, cough, and finally diarrhœa. (C, 11.)

LARYNX.—* Chronic dryness in the throat, and sensation of swelling in the larynx; and expectoration of thick mucus. (*Neidhard.*)

COUGH.—190. Slight cough.

Frequent slight cough, especially whilst eating. (*Husmann.* D, 16.)

In the evening tickling in the throat, with slight cough and headache.

Many evenings after lying down, a slight cough from tickling in the throat. (*Husmann.* D, 18.)

A dry cough, awakening him from sleep, which did not cease until he sat upright in bed, and flatus was discharged both upwards and downwards.

* Cough. (A, 16.)

* Continual severe cough, without expectoration, with pain in the breast, and circumscribed redness of the cheeks. (C. 14.)

195. * Tormenting cough, with expectoration; and circumscribed redness of the cheeks. (C. 13.)

* Feels stronger and freer in the breast in the mornings, and in the afternoon, and in the evening the customary dyspnœa does not appear. (*Husmann.* D, 18.)

A hot burning streaming in the right breast, begins under the right arm and clavicle, and draws itself downwards towards the region of the liver. (Afternoon of the third day. *Husmann.* D, 37.)

Acute stitches in the right breast in the region of the nipple. (*Husmann.* D, 39.)

* Pulmonary consumption. (A, 11, 14, 17.)

Aids expectoration. (A, 5, 17, 55.)

* Cough and expectoration. (C, 11.)

* Cough with coryza, then diarrhœa. (C, 11.)

200. * Croup. (A, 14, 15.)

BREAST.—Hooping cough. (A, 14, 17.)

* Hydrothorax. (A, 12.)

* Asthma. (A, 13.)

* Pneumonia. (A, 16, 17.)

205. * Typhoid pneumonia, with very difficult respiration, cheeks and hands lived, pulse full, soft, vibrating and easily compressed. (A, 18.)

* Diseases of the lungs. (A, 9, 10, 11, etc.)

* Pain in the breast, with periodic cough. (C, 12.)

* Pain in the breast, with cough and expectoration. C, 11.)

* Pain in the breast, with dry cough. (C, 14.)

* Burning and pressing in the breast, then heat through the abdomen and diarrhœa. (C, 16.)

Slowly shooting pain in the right side of the chest about the seventh rib. (*Jeanes*. D, 7.)

Acute stitch in the right breast.

Slowly shooting pain in the left side of the chest, near the axilla. (*Jeanes*. D, 6.)

210. Stitches from the lower part of the left breast to the shoulder.

Pressing pain in the region of the heart.

Stitches in the left side in the region of the short ribs, by moving and turning the body.

Constant pressure and heaviness in the whole of the upper part of the chest, with difficulty of breathing. (*Neidhard.*)

Slowly shooting pain under the sternum. (*Jeanes*. D, 5.)

Numb pain the whole length of the left scapula, along its inner edge, which is also increased by breathing. (*Neidhard.*)

Pressing pain in the breast and back.

215. Palpitation of the heart. (A, 48.) From immoderate doses, with great weakness. (A, 63.)

Stitches in both breasts.

Severe soreness under the right nipple, aggravated by being touched.

The nipples are sore and painful.

BACK.—220. Pain in the nape of the neck.

Soreness of the nape of the neck on being touched.

Pain in the left side of the nape of the neck.

Pain in the right side of the neck, as if sprained. (K. §.)

Stiffness of the nape of the neck. (*Bute*, 19.)

225. Pain in the back. (C, 20.)

Pain in the sacrum and bowels. (*Bute*, 150.)

* Pain in the sacrum from lifting. (C, 21.)

Pain in the sacrum which is alleviated by bending forward. (*Husmann*. D, 29.)

Rheumatic pains in the nape of the neck, shoulders and arms.

Pains in both shoulders.

230. Severe pain in the left shoulder, in the evenings.

Pain under the shoulder blade with chill. (*Bute*, 282.)

Pains from the left breast to the shoulder. (*Bute*, 210.)

Rheumatic pain in the right shoulder, worse in the forenoon, when she has retained the arm for a long time in the same position, drawing itself downwards to the elbow. (*Husmann*. D, 14.)

Pain on the top of the right shoulder. (*Husmann*. D, 28.)

Sudden rheumatic pains in the shoulder joint.

In the upper part of the shoulder joint severe pain in every motion.

235. * Rheumatic pain in the right arm and shoulder, worse at night in bed; cannot raise the arm. (C, 18.)

* Pain in the right shoulder, and in the upper part of the right arm, worse at night on turning in bed. (*Jeanes*.)

SUPERIOR EXTREMITIES.—Rheumatic pains in the arms and hands.

Rheumatic pains in the right fore arm in the evening.

Severe pain in the hand, with aching in the arm when lying warm and quiet in bed; it is also often felt in the left foot, now above, then in the instep, and then in the toes. (K.)

240. In the right palm near the index finger, a severe pain as from a bile.

* Burning of the palms. (C, 8.)

Redness of the hands and severe burning.

* Lividity of the hands in pneumonia. (A, 18.)

Numb pain in ball of the right thumb.

245. Cutting pain on the second joint of the left middle finger.

Sticking in the point of the right small finger.

Stiffness of the finger joints. (C, 7.)

Pain as from a bile at the root of the right thumb nail, then in the left, from this to all the fingers, one after another from the thumb to the small finger, alike on both hands.

250. * Ulceration at the roots of the nails, on all the fingers of both hands. (C, 22.)

INFERIOR EXTREMITIES.—Rheumatic pain in the left hip.

Pain as from a bruise in the left hip joint, whilst walk ing, but worse on rising from a seat.

* A rheumatic pain on the inside of the right thigh. (C, 17.)

* A bruise-like pain in the thigh, alternating with burning and pressure in the breast. (C, 16.)

* Stiffness of the knees. (C, 7.)

Stiffness and tightness in the bend and sides of the knees. (The fourth day. *Husmann*. D, 38.)

Cramp and pain in the calf of the left leg. (*Jeanes*.)

Drawing in the calves and into the instep, worse right than left. (*Husmann*. D, 27.)

Sticking pain in the right ankle.

Continual stitches under the right exterior ankle bone as from the sting of a bee.

Pain in the left foot with headache, (*Bute*, 18,) and during the pain in the right arm. (*Bute*, 139.)

Sticking as from a needle in the instep, in the morning in bed, and in the afternoon coldness of the feet. (C.7.)

260. Burning in the soles of the feet, and in the palms of the hands, forenoon.

Burning in the soles of the feet worse at night.

* Burning of the hands and feet, in the night. (C, 9.)

Pain in the corns.

Great weakness of the limbs, with pains in the sacrum, (The second day. *Husmann*. D, 29,) whilst walking. (*Husmann*. D, 33.)

LIMBS.—Rheumatic pains in the limbs.

* Acute, inflammatory, and arthritic rheumatism. (A, 22, 52.)

265. * (Acute swelling of the joints of the extremities.) (C, 19.)

Stiffness of the limbs and rheumatic pains, with headache. (*Bute*, 19.)

Pain in those places where the bones are least covered with flesh, but not in the joints; on touching the painful part, the pain immediately vanished and appeared in some other part. (Evening, 10 o'clock.)

GENERAL.—Great weakness. (*Bute.*)

Great prostration of muscular strength, by large doses. (A, 63.)

Extreme weakness and debility in the limbs, whilst walking in the open air. (Evening of the first day. *Husmann.* D, 21.)

Debility with vertigo and pain in the hypochondria. (*Bute*, 138.)

270. Great weakness, with the vomiting. (And afterwards. A, 39.)

Great weakness with suppression of the pulse. (A, 38,) with irregular pulse. (A, 63.)

Weakness and palpitation of the heart. (A, 48, 63.)

* Is tonic in diseases of the lungs. (A, 10.)

A quickly diffused and transient, but at the same time a very peculiar nervous thrill, which is often extended to the minutest extremity. (A, 61.)

A slowly shooting pain with long continued thrill, ending in a grumbling aching, in a carious molar tooth of the upper jaw. (*Jeanes.* D, 12.)

Fainting weakness. (A, 38, 40, 63.)

General sensitiveness and weakness.

Torpor and languor, from the seeds. (A, 46.)

* Paralysis of the right side of fourteen years duration, cured by the tincture in the dose of a small teaspoonful every three or four days. (Verbally from Dr. *B. Becker.*)

Convulsive rigidity of the limbs. (A, 63.)

SLEEP.—Sleeplessness at night.

He awakens at night with affright, as if he would fall.

Dreams two nights in succession of sailing on the sea.

280. Dreams, of a frightful and disagreeable character.

He awakens earlier than common. (*Husmann.* D, 19.)

FEVER.—In the evening in bed, chill and shivering in the back.

Shaking chill, with pain under the shoulder blade on motion.

Chill, with the headache. (*Bute.* 12, 22, 23.)

Chill and nausea. (*Bute.* 116.)

Transient feeling of heat before the regurgitation. (*Bute.* 7.)

Heat flying from the head to the stomach. (*Bute.* 29.)

* Sensation as if hot water was poured from the breast into the abdomen. (C, 56.)

Fever and delirium, from the seed. (A, 47.)

Burning heat, rapidly alternating with chill and shivering.

Abates irritative hardness and frequency of the pulse, also heat and dryness of the skin. (A, 59, 60.)

290. Pulsation through the whole body.

Rapid pulse.

A gradual increase in the force and fulness of the pulse: from moderate doses. (A, 54.)

The pulse rendered more frequent, by large emetic doses. (A, 37.)

Quickened circulation, with the vomiting. (A, 42.)

The frequency of the pulse diminished by the nausea. (A, 40.)

The frequency of the pulse diminished by small doses. (A, 42.)

Strength and frequency of the pulse extremely reduced, with irregularity, and with insensibility, coldness, &c., from very large doses. (A, 63.)

* Brings the pulse from 112 to 80. (A, 17.)

* Pulse full, soft and easily compressed, in pneumonia. (A, 18.)

Suppression of the pulse, with fainting, from large doses. (A, 37, 63.)

Seeds have great influence on the pulse. (A, 45.)

SKIN.—Heat and dryness of the skin. (A, 60.)

Increased itching, of an old tubercle-like eruption on the skin.

305. * Itching and nettle-rash before the nausea. (C, 23.)

* Warts. (A, 26.)

* Old indolent ulcers; ill conditional ulcers with callous borders, and ichorous discharge. (A, 27, 28.)

* Nasal polypi: fungous excrescences, &c. (A, 29, 32.)

GENERAL.—Constant change of the symptoms, when a new one arises the earlier cease.

310. The most of the symptoms appear to be aggravated in the evenings and mornings.

* Diaphoretic. (A, 2, 5, 17, 25, 41.)

* Intermittent fever, marsh fever, nervous fever. (A, 23, 24.)

* Jaundice. (A, 6, 7, 8.)

C.—*Curative operations observed by Dr. G. H. Bute.*

1. Vertigo by quickly turning the head, or by looking upward.
2. Distension of the temporal veins, which were painfully sensitive to the touch.
3. Feeling of soreness on small spots on the head, especially in the temples.
4. Several cases of angina, especially a form of pharyngitis.
5. Hæmorrhoids.
6. A female who had distension of abdomen in the evening, and flatulent discharges, per vaginam, from the os uteri, which was constantly open, at the same time a pain passing in rays from the nape of the neck into the head.
7. In a lady; coldness of the feet in the afternoons, at the same time the tongue was painful and sore upon being touched, like a bile; and there was stiffness of the knee and finger joints.
8. Burning of the palms of the hands and soles of

the feet, compelling to throw the bed clothes off the feet, for the purpose of cooling them. In many cases of ladies in the climacteric years.

9. Burning of the hands and feet at night.

10. Burning of the ears, with a redness of one cheek.

11. In a man of scrofulous habit; after taking cold, coryza, then rawness of the throat, then pain in the breast, with cough and expectoration, and finally diarrhœa.

12. Pain in the breast, with periodic cough.

13. Tormenting cough and expectoration, with circumscribed redness of the cheeks.

14. In an unmarried lady of thirty years of age; constant severe cough, without expectoration, with pain in the breast, and circumscribed redness of the cheeks. A dose removed the cough for an hour, and many repeated doses perfectly removed the disease.

15. In a lady; pain in the left hypochondrium, which was rendered worse by coughing, but was better from being pressed, and by lying towards the left side; very copious urination at night.

16. In a man; for some years very frequent attacks of burning and pressure in the breast, which alternated with a bruise-like pain in the thigh, but never appearing in both places at the same time. The affection of the breast always ended with the feeling as if hot water poured itself from the chest into the abdomen, which was followed by diarrhœal stools.

17. Many kinds of arthritic and rheumatic pains; pain in the inner side of the right thigh, like rheumatism, &c. &c.

18. Rheumatic pain in the right arm and shoulder, worse at night in bed, so that the arm could not be raised; of a year's duration, perfectly cured.

19. In a case of gout, with very considerable tumefaction of the joints of all the extremities; obvious displacement of the right shoulder and shoulder-blade;

cramp in the nape of the neck and in the larynx, and bad taste in the mouth, the sanguinaria was of great service.

20. Several cases of pain in the back.

21. Pain in the loins, caused suddenly by lifting.

22. Ulceration at the roots of all the nails of both hands, in a young man, who had just arrived from a long sea voyage.

23. General itching in the skin, with a disposition to nettle-rash, preceded by nausea.

24. It appears to be an important remedy in scarlatina.

D.

Doctor *Jeanes*, after decanting the tincture of the root of the sanguinaria, and preparing the first and second dilutions, observing that he was affected with nausea, noted that, and the accompanying symptoms which follow:

1. Nausea, as if vomiting was about to take place; as after taking a disagreeable purgative medicine; and a feeling as if diarrhœa was about to occur.

2. A slowly shooting pain in the left ear.

3. Cramp and pain in the calf of the left leg.

4. A pain in the forehead, of the same character as that in the ear.

5. A similar pain under the sternum.

6. A similar pain in the left side of the chest near the axilla.

7. A similar pain in the right side of the chest, about the seventh rib.

8. A transitory and slight, but peculiar sensation in the fauces, as if something acrimonious had been swallowed.

9. Discharge of flatus, then of excrementitious matter, with abatement of the nausea, &c.

10. A prickling sensation in the tongue and roof of the mouth, as after chewing mezereum, but slighter.

11. Pain in one or more of the incisor teeth, and in a decayed molar tooth.

12. A slowly shooting and thrilling pain in a carious molar tooth of the upper jaw, which passed off gradually in that form of pain which is often termed a grumbling tooth-ache.

Doctor *F. Husmann* made the following experiments with sanguinaria. Some pellets of the sixth potence were taken in the evening and in the following morning by J. H. and F. H. Neither of them knew the symptoms which were already attributed to this agent, nor those which were produced in each other, until these had been written. The following were observed in J. H.

13. On awaking in the morning, a crawling feeling on the point of the tongue, and an acrid sensation which extended itself over the whole tongue.

14. Rheumatic pain in the right shoulder, worse in the forenoon, when she had retained the arm long in the same position, drawing itself down into the elbow.

15. Awakes with pain in a carious tooth in the right upper jaw, and pain in the right side of the forehead, and extending to the ear; the tooth-ache was aggravated by cold water, (and also by hot drinking,) but better by warm water.

16. Frequent hacking cough whilst eating, for many days.

17. On the seventh day the menses appeared at their proper time, but very copious, much more so than commonly, yet with less sacral pain and weakness than usual; but on the other hand with pain in the right side of the forehead and head, accompanied by a feeling as if the eyes would press out of the head, worse on the right side.

18. Many evenings after lying down a hacking cough from tickling in the throat.

The following symptoms were observed by F. H.

19. Prickling in the tip of the tongue, in fifteen minutes after taking.

20. Next morning, immediately after awaking, a feeling of dryness and rawness, such as occurs after acrid things, beginning on the right side of the tongue, then extending itself over the whole tongue.

21. In the morning of the first day he feels stronger and freer in the breast; and a difficulty of breathing, which he has felt every afternoon and evening for fourteen days, does not occur.

22. He awakes earlier than common.

23. The first day, two stools.

24. In the evening of the first day, whilst walking in the open air, extremely weak and debilitated in the lower extremities.

25. Transient pain of the right side of the forehead, like a pressing, only whilst standing still; better whilst walking.

26. Pain deep in the left ear, only for a short time, during the pain in the forehead.

27. Pain in a carious molar tooth, in the right lower jaw, after cold drinking; two mornings in succession.

28. In the afternoons pain in the fore part of the head as from fulness.

29. Pressing above on the head, and in the region of the anterior fontanelle; disappears whilst walking.

30. Drawing in the calves of the legs and into the instep, worse in the right than the left.

31. Pain in the top of the right shoulder.

32. The second day, great weakness in the lower limbs, and pain in the loins, relieved by bending forward.

33. On the third day he remarked that by drawing the tips of the fingers lightly over the right cheek, a crackling was felt in the ear of that side; this was not the case with the left.

34. In the afternoon, about two o'clock, a feeling in the eyes, as if they were exposed to acid vapor.

35. Hiccough whilst smoking tobacco.

36. Very weak in the lower limbs whilst walking.

37. Sticking on the left side of the tongue.

38. Heat in the throat, the inspiration of cool air is pleasant, and alleviates the sensation. In the evening from six to seven o'clock.

39. Boring pain above in the fore part of the head.

40. A hot burning streaming in the right breast; it begins under the right arm and clavicle and draws downwards towards the region of the liver. In the afternoon.

41. The fourth day. Stiffness and drawing in the bend and sides of the knees.

42. Acute stitches in the right breast, in the region of the nipple.

43. Seminal emissions two nights in succession, (between the 6th and 8th days,) after which he feels very well.

44. The eighth day, in the afternoon, a twisting pain above the groin, on the left side, equi-distant from the symphysis pubis, and the crista illi; worse whilst sitting, standing or bending to the right side; increased by pressure; better whilst walking erect. The pain after a time went from this spot around to the left hip, and then upwards to the back on the short ribs.

45. The first day soft stool, the later days rather costive.

TRIOSTEUM* PERFOLIATUM.

BY W. WILLIAMSON, M. D.

Synon. T. majus, — T. floribus verticillatis sessilibus,—T. foliis connatis, floribus sessilibus verticillatis. —Breitblättriger Dreystein.

Vulgo. Dr. Tinker's weed, Wild Coffee, Gentian, Horse Gentian, White Gentian, Horse Ginseng, Fever Root, Fever Wort, Wild Ipecac, Bastard Ipecacuanha, Sweet Bitter, Cinque, &c.

Nat. Syst. Juss. Caprifoliaceæ.

Nat. Ord. Lin. Aggregatæ.

Class. Pentandria.

Order. Monogynia.

GEN. CHAR. *Calyx* persistent, dark purple, five-cleft, segments of the length of the corolla, linear, acute.

Corol. Tubular, five-lobed, sub-equal, gibbous at the base.

Stam. Included.

Stig. Capitate, sub-five-lobed.

Berry. Three-celled, three-seeded and crowned with the calyx.

The flowers resemble those of the sweet scented shrub in appearance.

SPEC. CHAR. *Leaves* large oval, acuminate, abruptly narrowed at the base, connate, sub-pubescent beneath, the two uppermost pairs are small and convoluted till after the inflorescence is past, when they become developed to the full size and assume a brownish purple colour. *Flowers* axillary, sessile and whorled in triplets, three, six or nine around the stem ; blooms in the latter

* Three bony seeds.

end of May. *Corolla* reddish purple above, striated below and pubescent. The *berries* are ovate, commonly six in a whorl, sometimes purple, but generally of an orange colour; they have three divisions, each containing one hard seed, and ripen in September.

The plant inhabits rich hilly woodlands, and the edge of cultivated grounds, and grows from two to four feet high, several stalks arising from the same root. The stems are about three-eighths of an inch in diameter, simple, erect, cylindrical, pubescent and of a green colour. The root is perennial, contorted, tuberculated or gibbous, of a brownish colour, giving off horizontal branches from eighteen inches to two feet in length, about the size of the finger in diameter, yellowish externally and whitish internally.

From pharmaceutical experiments, it has been observed that when the plant is treated with water it yields a larger quantity of active extract, than when treated with alcohol, and that the alcoholic extract is perfectly soluble in water, proving that the medicinal properties of the triosteum do not consist of resinous matter. The active principle cannot be obtained by distillation. The leaves yield the largest quantity of soluble matter, but that obtained from the root possesses the greatest activity.

Both the leaves and the root of the triosteum are quite bitter to the taste. The root is also nauseous to the taste, and has an odour somewhat resembling ipecacuanha.

The medicinal properties of the triosteum, allœopathically considered, are four-fold, viz: emetic, cathartic, diaphoretic and diuretic, and by some, if given in small doses, a tonic. The larger doses, and especially when prepared from the bark of the root, are found to act with great certainty and energy on the alimentary canal, both by emesis and catharsis, while a decoction of the leaves are found to produce merely a diaphoretic effect.

When kept in the dry state, its medicinal properties are said to be very much impaired by age.

The berries, after being dried and roasted, have been

used by the settlers of the interior of the country, as a substitute for coffee, and hence, one of its common names—wild coffee. It has been recommended by old school practitioners, as an emectic in intermittent fevers and pleurisy.

The Triosteum perfoliatum held a high rank in the Materia Medica of some tribes of Indians in this country, as we learn from that excellent Botanist, Dr. Wm. Darlington, who well recollects the last *Indian Doctress* of the Delaware tribe, in the vicinity of West Chester, who seemed to consider it a sort of panacea, and prescribed it in all cases of disease, without distinction.

The following symptoms were obtained from taking a few drops of the tincture in water, every day, for three successive days.

Dulness and drowsiness, with disinclination to engage actively in business.

Greater cheerfulness. (First day. *Neidhard.*)

Sleepiness without the ability to sleep sound after midnight.

SKIN.—Vesicular eruption on the forehead over the left eye, on the middle of the chest and on the right arm. (*Neidhard.*)

5. Very great itching at night, with welts all over the surface. (*Neidhard.*)

Violent itching eruption of the skin, generally with elevation of the skin. (Second day. *Neidhard.*)

FEVER.—General perspiration.

Drying away of the perspiration, and development of fever, with hot skin and increased thirst.

Aching in all the bones.

HEAD.—10. Giddiness when rising at midnight, with extreme drowsiness.

Headache which is worse in the right side of the fore part of the head, and right temple.

Pain in the hinder part of the head with the sensation of weight.

Increasing pain in the head.

Headache worse from sitting up.

15. Boring pain in the left temple.

Boring pain in the right temple, at 3 o'clock, A. M.

Pain in the right side of the head and in the back. (47.)

Pain in the nape and occiput, with coldness and stiffness in the feet. (58.)

EYES.—Slight pain in the left eye-ball.

NOSE.—20. Sneezing.

THROAT.—Soreness as if from swelling of the pharynx, and pain in the œsophagus on swallowing. (*Neidhard.*)

APPETITE.—Increased appetite through the day.

Loathing of all food.

Thirst but not a very urgent desire for drink.

STOMACH.—25. At 4 o'clock in the morning, the feeling of a load and oppression in the epigastrium, with throbbing and an undulating sensation all through the system.

Pain in the epigastrium increased by drinking water.

Pain in the epigastrium increased by turning in bed.

Oppression in the epigastrium through the night.

Soreness in the epigastric region. (*Neidhard.*)

30. Slight nausea.

Nausea on rising, which was immediately followed by copious vomiting of very sour ingesta, attended with cramp in the stomach, and followed by perspiration and a pain in the forehead, which was worse on the left side.

Vomiting at 5 o'clock in the morning on rising to stool.

Vomiturition, attended with severe pain in the epigastrium, and drawing in the calves of the legs, almost amounting to a cramp. (56.)

Flatulency, confined to the stomach.

35. Heat and sharp pain in the right side of the abdomen in the evening.

BOWELS.—Stool at 7 o'clock, A. M., followed by numbness of the lower extremities. (56.)

Copious evacuation of thin stools from the bowels, without pain.

The evacuations from the bowels seemed to proceed from the small intestines.

Stools watery or frothy, voided without pain, and are followed by exhaustion.

40. Evacuation from the bowels, at 7 o'clock, A. M., preceded by pain in the abdomen.

The evacuations are most frequent in the evening.

* A diarrhœa attended with colic pains. (*Neidhard.*)

Irritation in the anus with exudation of mucus. (*Neidhard.*)

GENITALS.—Discharge of semen during sleep without erection.

CHEST AND HEART.—45. Audible beating of the heart and slight pain under the left breast.

TRUNK.—Pain in the right shoulder from lying on it.

Pain in the nape and back. (17.)

Pain in the nape with perspiration.

Rheumatic pain in the back from stooping.

50. Pain and stiffness in the loins.

The pain in the loins is confined to the left side.

EXTREMITIES.—Stiffness of all the joints of the upper, as well as of the lower extremities.

Remarkable stiffness in the lower extremities with slight coldness, and a tingling sensation.

Stiffness in the knees when attempting to rise.

55. Pain in the right knee.

Numbness in the calves of the legs. (36, 33.)

Penetrating pain under and behind the left external malleolus after sleeping.

Stiffness of the joints of the toes, ankles and knees when lying. (18.)

Drawing and shrinking sensation in the legs, and the most decided pricking in the soles or the feet.

Coldness and stiffness in the feet. (18.)

REPERTORIUM.

GENERAL EFFECTS.

Chills, down the back with heat in the st., Lob. i.
Cold, greater ability to bear it. Oxal. ac.
Consciousness, loss of. Oxal. ac.
Convulsions, just before or at the time of death. Oxal. ac.
Debility, general, Eup. p., Lob. i.
Dislocated, sens. as if the shoulder and hip joints would be. Fluor. ac.
Erratic pain, slight, in left half of the body, with slight itching. Fluor. ac.
Influenza of old people and inebriates. Eup. p.
——— with weakness of the pulse, and great general prostration. Eup. p.
Intermitting symptoms. Oxal. ac.
Jerking pain in different parts of the body, behind the left ear, on left middle finger, in Os. sacrum, &c. Fluor. ac.
——— burning pains, violent, confined to a small space. Fluor. ac.
——— pains, sudden shocks of. Pod. p.
Joints, affections of. Oxal. ac.
Lameness, sens. of, and pressure in the hand, arm, foot, &c. Fluor. ac.
Languor, excessive. Fluor. ac., Oxal. ac.
Morning, aggravation of symptoms. Pod. p.
——— feeling as from previous debauch. Oxal. ac.
Motion, of different parts, as feet, hands, eyelids, facial muscles, &c. Fluor. ac.
——— singularly easy. Fluor. ac.
Neuralgia, Elat.
Numbness, gen., approaching palsy. Oxal. ac.
Pains, aching, in the bones of the fore arms and legs. Fluor. ac.
—— aggravated by movement. Oxal. ac.
—— of short duration, in left leg, arm and hand. Fluor. ac.
—— chiefly affecting the left side. Elat.

Pains occupying but a small spot, half an inch to an inch in length. Fluor. ac.
—— sharp, fugitive, or dull aching shifting. Elat.
Pressing pain in different parts in the evening. Fluor. ac.
Rheumatism, accompanied by perspiration and soreness of the bones. Eup. p.
Shivering, through the whole body. Lob. i.
Sitting, whilst, pleasurable movements of the whole body. Fluor. ac.
Symptoms, aggravated, evening and morning. Sang. c.
—— aggravated in the morning, better in the evening. Pod. p.
—— constant change of. Sang. c.
Tired easily, in the evening. Fluor. ac.
Tremor, of the limbs. Oxal. ac.
Walking, difficult. Fluor. ac.
Weakness, and numbness in limbs and back. Oxal. ac.

MENTAL AFFECTIONS.

Anger. Fluor. ac.
Anxiety. Fluor. ac.
Apathy. Fluor. ac.
Aversion, to conversation. Oxal. ac.
—— to business. Fluor. ac.
—— to exercise. Kalm. l.
Cheerfulness, excessive. Fluor. ac.
Concentration of mind, unusual. Oxal. ac.
Contentment, perfect. Fluor. ac.
Dejection. Elat., Eup. p.
Displeased, easily. Fluor. ac.
Discontentedness, in the evening. Fluor. ac.
Fear of some approaching disaster. Elat.
Forgetfulness of the most common occurrences. Fluor. ac.
—— in business. Fluor. ac.
—— of dates. Fluor. ac.
Fury. Fluor ac.
Gaiety of mind excessive, in the morning. Fluor. ac.
Hatred of absent persons, disappearing as soon as they are seen. Fluor. ac.
Hilarity. Fluor. ac., Oxal. ac.
Horror, ideas of. Fluor. ac.
Inattention. Fluor. ac.
Ill humor. Fluor. ac.
Illusions, of the senses. Fluor. ac.
Indifference to dangers which appear to menace one. Fluor. ac.

Irritability, towards evening, which continues next morning. Kalm. l.
Love of children excessive. Oxal. ac.
Meditation, difficult and slow in the morning. Oxal. ac.
Merriment, excessive. Oxal. ac.
Moroseness. Sang. c.
Sing, disposition to. Lob. c.
Talk, disinclination to. Oxal. ac.
Thoughts, active. Oxal. ac.

SLEEP, ETC.

Awaking at midnight. Benz. ac.
——— at 2 o'clock, A. M., from strong internal heat and hard bounding pulse. Benz. ac.
——— earlier than usual. Sang. c
——— after midnight, with violent pulsation of the heart and temporal arteries, and cannot fall asleep again. Benz. ac.
Dreams, anxious. Lob. i.
——— disagreeable but not vexatious. Fluor. ac.
——— fantastic. Kalm. l.
——— frightful. Sang. c., Fluor. ac.
——— lascivious. Oxal. ac.
——— lucid. Fluor. ac.
——— unpleasant. Oxal. ac., Kalm. l., Sang. c.
——— vivid. Fluor. ac., Oxal. ac.
——— sad. Lob. i.
——— of dying. Fluor. ac.
——— of distant acquaintances and things. Fluor. ac.
——— of sudden death of friends. Fluor. ac.
——— of rapid sliding walking. Oxal. ac.
——— of sailing on the sea, two nights in succession. Sang. c
——— of water being poured on one. Oxal. ac.
——— unable to remember. Fluor. ac., Oxal. ac.
——— with frequent waking. Oxal. ac.
——— towards morning, of a frightful character. Fluor. ac.
Gaping, incessant. Elat.
Sleeplessness. Fluor. ac., Oxal. ac., Sang. c.
——— day and night. Fluor. ac.
——— in the evening. Fluor. ac.
——— at night. Sang. c.
——— after midnight. Sang. c.
Sleep, profound. Fluor. ac., Oxal. ac.
——— restless. Kalm. l., Lob. i., Oxal. ac.
——— starting in, with jerking of the hands. Lob. c.

Sleep, talking in. Kalm. l.
—— walking in. Kalm. l.
—— with snoring. Fluor. ac.
—— with sobbing. Lob. i.
—— with anxious, frightful dreams, and awaking at midnight. Fluor. ac.
Yawning, violent. Oxal ać.

FEBRILE AFFECTIONS.

Fevers, bilious, with colic, and watery discharges from the bowels. Elat.
—— exhausting, with dyspepsia and hiccough. Oxal. ac.
—— evening. Sang. c.
Fever, *Intermittent*. Elat., Eup. p., Pod. p.
—— —— quotidian. Elat., Eup. p., Pod. p.
—— —— quartan. Elat., Eup. p., Pod. p.
—— —— tertian. Elat., Eup. p., Pod. p.
—— —— attended with thirst, throughout the night before the paroxysm. Eup. p.
—— —— attended by,
—— —— aching pain and moaning throughout the cold stage. Eup. p.
—— —— distressing pain in the scrobiculus cordis, throughout the chill and heat. Eup. p.
—— —— a heavy chill in the morning of one day, and about noon the next. Eup. p.
—— —— cough in the night previous to the paroxysm. Eup. p.
—— —— (loose) in the intermission. Eup. p.
—— —— throbbing headache, during the chill and heat. Eup. p.
—— —— vomiting at the conclusion of the chill. Eup. p.
—— —— pain in abd., and watery evacuations from the bowels. Elat.
—— —— loss of appetite during the apyrexia. Pod. p.
—— —— delirium and loquacity, during the hot stage, with forgetfulness afterwards of all that passed. Pod. p.
—— —— vomiting of bile at the close of the hot stage. Eup. p.
—— —— thirst during the chill, and heat with vomiting after each draught of water. Eup. p.
—— —— worse in the morning of one day and afternoon of the next, Eup. p.
—— —— followed by little or no perspiration. Eup. p.

Fever, attended by,
—— constipation. Pod. p.
—— dry, hot skin. Eup. p., Trios.
—— delirium. Pod. p.
—— aching of the bones of the extremities, and soreness of the flesh. Eup. p.
—— aching of all the bones. Trios. p.
—— aching pain, and soreness as if from having been beaten in the calves of the legs, small of back and arms. Eup. p.
—— flushed face. Eup. p.
—— retching and vomiting of bile. Eup. p.
—— coldness, trembling and nausea. Eup. p.
—— internal trembling and external heat. Eup. p.
—— pain in the morning before the paroxysm. Eup. p.
—— *diarrhœa*. Elat.
—— violent headache and thirst. Pod. p.
—— chill in the morning at 7 o'clock, with pressing pain in both hypochondria, and dull aching pains in the knees and ankles, elbows and wrists. Pod. p.
—— thirst. Pod. p.
—— sens.! as if hot water was poured from the breast into the abdomen. Sang. c.
—— sleep and moaning. Eup. p.
—— soreness of the bones. Eup. p.
—— vomiting after every draught. Eup. p.
—— despondency, morbid sensitiveness of the skin, and sleeplessness. Eup. p.
—— alternate chilliness, and flashes of heat. Eup. p.
—— trembling in the back. Eup. p.
—— sleeplessness. Eup. p.
—— followed by,
—— great lassitude. Eup. p.
—— slight perspiration. Eup. p.
—— forgetfulness of words. Pod. p.
—— preceded by,
—— cold and shivering on two successive days. Kalm. l.
—— chill and shivering in the back, in the evening. Sang. c.
Chills, in the morning. Eup. p., Pod. p.
—— at 9 o'clock. Eup. p.
—— at 7 o'clock, preceded by thirst, and attended by moisture of the hands. Eup. p.
—— in the evening, with sneezing. Eup. p.
—— hastened by drinking cold water. Eup. p.
—— after the vomiting. Eup. p.
—— attended by, headache. Eup. p., Pod. p., Sang c
—— backache and thirst. Eup. p.

Chills, nausea. Sang. c., Eup. p.
—— coldness and stinging or pricking in the feet. Eup. p.
—— unusual shivering. Eup. p.
—— stiffness of the fingers. Eup. p.
—— shaking, and pain under the shoulder-blade on motion. Sang. c.
Chills, preceded by,
—— pain in the back. Pod. p., Eup. p.
—— pain above the right ilium with thirst and yawning. Eup. p.
—— violent pains in the head and back. Eup. p.
—— followed by,
—— nausea and vomiting. Eup. p.
Chilliness.
—— in the morning. Eup. p.
—— from motion. Eup. p.
—— through the night and in the morning, with nausea. Eup. p.
Chilliness, attended by,
———— Gaping. Elat.
———— nausea. Eup. p.
———— trembling and nausea. Eup. p.
———— thirst. Eup. p.
Coldness, during nocturnal perspiration. Eup. p.
Heat, gen.
—— after exercise. Fluor. ac.
—— sens. of. Oxal. ac.
—— sens. as if a burning vapour was emitted from the pores of the whole body. Fluor. ac.
—— flushes of.
—— ———— with perspiration. Oxal. ac.
—— in the evening.
—— sens. of increased warmth. Fluor. ac.
—— forenoon.
—— sens. of internal, particularly in the face. Oxal. ac.
—— first in the face, then in the left leg, as from external warmth. Oxal. ac.
—— pungent during the nocturnal perspiration. Eup. p.
Heat, attended by,
—— aching of the bones of the extremities. Eup. p.
—— delirium and loquacity. Pod. p.
—— nausea and sickness. Eup. p.
—— headache and trembling. Eup. p.
—— increased headache, but diminished thirst Eup p
—— throbbing headache. Eup. p.
—— thirst. Pod. p., Trios.
—— followed by,
—— little or no perspiration. Eup. p.

Perspiration, clammy. Oxal. ac.
——— cold. Eup. p.
——— —— of hands, feet and face. Oxal. ac.
——— profuse, of hands, feet and face. Fluor. ac.
——— diminished. Eup. p., Oxal. ac.
——— glutinous, with itching. Fluor. ac.
——— nocturnal. Eup. p., Pod. p.
——— sour. Fluor. ac.
——— in the evening. Eup. p., Fluor. ac.
——— —— offensive. Fluor. ac.
——— —— slight. Eup. p.
——— gen. Trios.
——— accompanied by,
——— sens. of heat, on the upper part of the body, towards the right. Fluor. ac.
——— cold creepings, particularly from the lower part of the spine upwards. Oxal. ac.

Pulse, accelerated. Oxal. ac., Sang. c.
—— diminished. Sang. c.
—— frequent. Oxal. ac., Sang. c.
—— full. Sang. c.
—— hard. Oxal. ac., Sang. c.
—— quick. Sang. c.
—— imperceptible. Oxal. ac.
—— intermittent. Oxal. ac.
—— irregular. Sang. c.
—— quick. Sang. c.
—— rapid. Sang. c.
—— slow. Kalm. l., Pod. p., Sang. c.
—— small. Sang. c.
—— soft. Sang. c.
—— suppressed. Sang. c.
—— tense. Oxal. ac.
—— tremulous. Oxal. ac.
—— ——— with coldness, clammy sweats and lividity of finger nails. Oxal. ac.
—— fainting. Sang. c.
—— coldness and insensibility. Sang. c.

SKIN, ETC.

Blotches, on the skin.
——— red, elevated, above the eyebrows. Fluor. ac.
Blood-vesicles, small, light red, round, elevated, mostly on the right side, disappearing for a moment after strong pressure. Fluor. ac.
Burning pains on small spots of the skin. Fluor. ac.
——— —— angle of the index finger. Fluor. ac.

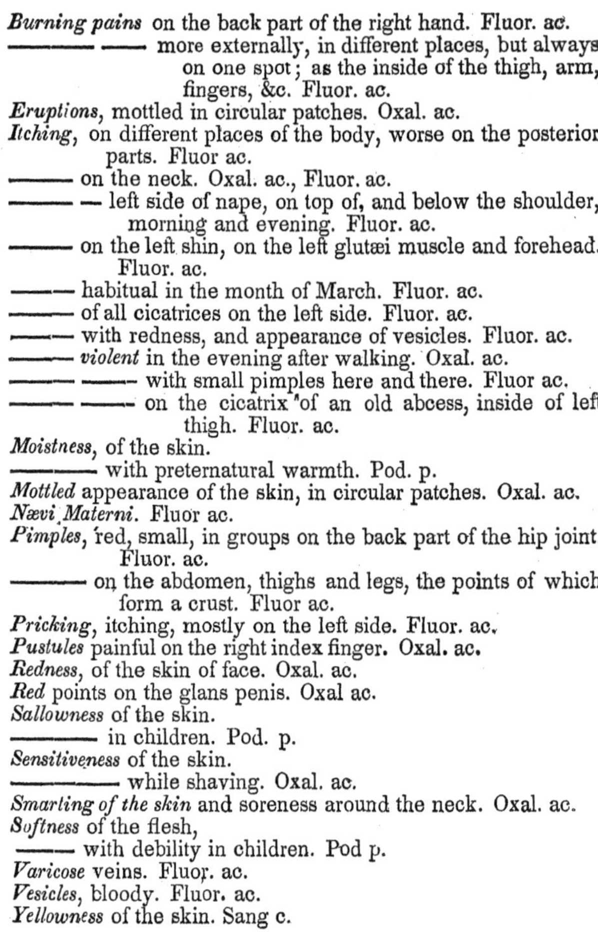

Burning pains on the back part of the right hand. Fluor. ac.

——— —— more externally, in different places, but always on one spot; as the inside of the thigh, arm, fingers, &c. Fluor. ac.

Eruptions, mottled in circular patches. Oxal. ac.

Itching, on different places of the body, worse on the posterior parts. Fluor ac.

——— on the neck. Oxal. ac., Fluor. ac.

——— — left side of nape, on top of, and below the shoulder, morning and evening. Fluor. ac.

——— on the left shin, on the left glutæi muscle and forehead. Fluor. ac.

——— habitual in the month of March. Fluor. ac.

——— of all cicatrices on the left side. Fluor. ac.

——— with redness, and appearance of vesicles. Fluor. ac.

——— *violent* in the evening after walking. Oxal. ac.

——— ——— with small pimples here and there. Fluor ac.

——— ——— on the cicatrix of an old abcess, inside of left thigh. Fluor. ac.

Moistness, of the skin.

——— with preternatural warmth. Pod. p.

Mottled appearance of the skin, in circular patches. Oxal. ac.

Nævi Materni. Fluor ac.

Pimples, red, small, in groups on the back part of the hip joint. Fluor. ac.

——— on the abdomen, thighs and legs, the points of which form a crust. Fluor ac.

Pricking, itching, mostly on the left side. Fluor. ac.

Pustules painful on the right index finger. Oxal. ac.

Redness, of the skin of face. Oxal. ac.

Red points on the glans penis. Oxal ac.

Sallowness of the skin.

——— in children. Pod. p.

Sensitiveness of the skin.

——— while shaving. Oxal. ac.

Smarting of the skin and soreness around the neck. Oxal. ac.

Softness of the flesh,

——— with debility in children. Pod p.

Varicose veins. Fluor. ac.

Vesicles, bloody. Fluor. ac.

Yellowness of the skin. Sang c.

HEAD.

Burning, first in forehead, afterwards in jaws, occiput and bladder. Fluor. ac.

Chilliness of the left side of head, with sens. as if the hair would raise on end. Lob. i.
Congestion of blood to the head. Fluor. ac., Sang. c.
——— sens. of, proceeding from the throat. Fluor. ac.
——— with whizzing in the ears, and sens. of heat. Sang. c.
Confusion of head, with drowsiness. Benz. ac.
Distress, on the top, and in the back part of head. Eup. p.
——— drawing pain in head and eyes. Kalm. l.
——— worse towards evening. Kalm. l.
Dulness of the head. Fluor. ac., Kalm. l., Lob. i., Pod. p., Sang. c.
——— of occiput. Fluor. ac.
——— ——— towards the right. Fluor. ac.
——— with painful tension towards the right. Fluor. ac.
——— with sleepiness in the morning. Pod. p.
——— in the evening. Kalm. l.
——— in the morning. Fluor. ac.
——— of occiput and forehead. Lob. i.
Dull pain in the region of causality. Elat.
——— in the region of combativeness. Elat.
——— pressure from the nape upwards, extending. Fluor. ac.
Emptiness of head, (hollowness) sens. of. Oxal. ac.
Forehead, boring pain in. Sang. c.
——— burning pain in. Fluor. ac.
——— compressing pain in right frontal protuberance. Fluor. ac.
——— congestion of blood to, like a quick jerk. Fluor. ac.
——— darting pain in. Sang. c.
——— ——— at night. Sang. c.
——— deep in the middle of, pain. Fluor. ac.
——— dull heavy pain in. Fluor. ac., Oxal. ac.
——— ——— with soreness over the seat of pain. Pod. p.
——— ——— passing round in a line above the eyebrows. Lob. i.
——— fulness above the eyes. Oxal. ac.
——— pain in. Sang. c.
——— pain in, as if it would split, with chill; and with burning in stomach. Sang. c.
——— pain in left frontal protuberance, worse in afternoon Pod. p.
——— pressing in. Kalm. l.
——— ——— with drawing. Sang. c.
——— ——— pain in, as if in the bone. Fluor. ac.
——— pulsating in. Kalm. l.
——— rending pain in. Kalm. l.

Forehead, right side of, pain. Fluor. ac., Sang. c., Trios
——— ——— better while moving. Sang. c.
——— left side of, pain. Fluor. ac.
——— slow shooting pain in. Sang. c.
——— shooting pains in left side of. Fluor. ac.
——— sudden pain in, with sore throat, in the evening. Pod. p.
——— and temples, pain. Fluor. ac., Kalm. l.
——— pain on the right side in evening. Sang. c.
——— and vertex, pain, towards the right. Fluor. ac.
——— every day, pain in. Kalm. l.
——— in the evening pain in. Fluor. ac., Kalm. l.
Headache, with nausea and vomiting. Lob. i.
——— to the left upper jaw, passing. Fluor. ac.
——— to the lower jaws, extending. Oxal. ac.
——— from the forehead to occiput, extending. Eup. p.
——— along the base of the occipital bone. Oxal. ac.
——— always drawing upward from the neck. Sang. c.
——— with heat in the face. Fluor. ac.
——— with chill. Sang. c.
——— between the vertex and occiput. Oxal. ac.
——— when lying down. Sang. c.
——— over the right eyebrow. Fluor. ac.
——— paroxysmal. Sang. c.
——— dull after dinner. Lob. i.
——— in right side of, and back. Trios.
——— alternating with diarrhœa. Pod. p.
——— from the anterior angle of right eye, to forehead, extending. Sang. c.
——— in all the left side of head, extending to the eye, with similar pain in the left foot. Sang. c.
——— with rheumatic pains and stiffness of the limbs and neck preceded by nausea. Sang. c.
Heat, in head and face. Pod. p.
Heaviness of the head. Fluor. ac., Kalm. l., Lob. i., Sang. c.
——— first in the right then in the left side. Kalm. l.
——— above the eyes. Fluor. ac.
——— worse on motion. Fluor. ac.
Heavy pain in the left half of the head. Fluor. ac.
Jerking, violent in the interior, behind and above the right eyebrow. Fluor. ac.
Looseness of brain, sens. of. Kalm. l.
Occiput, pain in. Eup. p., Fluor. ac., Lob. i., Trios.
——— aching. Fluor. ac.
——— dull. Fluor. ac., Kalm. l., Lob. i.
——— pressing. Fluor. ac., Lob. i.
——— sens. of soreness and beating. Eup. p.

Occiput, with sens. of weight after lying. Eup. p., Trios.
——— and nape, with stiffness. Trios.
Pressure inward. Oxal. ac.
——— in the occiput towards the right, with a sens. of numbness and pricking in the left forearm. Fluor. ac.
——— pain in right temple. Kalm. l.
——— outwards from within, sens. of. Fluor. ac.
Pressing pain in forehead and right eye on stooping. Fluor. ac.
——— upwards, sens. as if the brain was. Fluor. ac.
Rushing in the head. Kalm. l.
——— pain in forehead towards the left. Kalm. l.
——— ——— on rising from bed. Kalm. l.
——— ——— in right temple. Kalm. l.
——— in head and neck. Kalm. l.
——— of blood, sens. of across the head. Eup. p.
Rolling of h., during difficult dentition in children. Pod. p.
Shaking, gen., frequent sens. of, with a dull pressure and compression in the occiput, towards the right. Fluor. ac.
——— in the back part of head, towards the right, in the forenoon. Fluor. ac.
Shivering of h. sens. of, without coldness, passing from the top of the head to the neck. Kalm. l.
Shocks, from the nape towards the occiput. Kalm. l.
——— of pain sudden through the h. Lob. i.
Temples, pain in. Elat., Kalm. l.
——— darting pain in. Eup. p., Fluor. ac.
——— ——— in right t. Kalm. l.
——— dull pain in. Fluor. ac.
——— distension of veins in. Sang. c.
——— quick throbbing in. Fluor. ac.
——— jerking in. Oxal. ac.
——— soreness in, and pain in spots. Sang. c.
——— pressure in, from within outwards. Fluor. ac.
——— ——— with a dull pressing in the flesh above the left elbow, and hands feel paralyzed. Lob. i.
——— shooting pain in. Fluor. ac., Lob. i.
——— stunning, relieved by pressure. Pod. p.
——— soreness in right parietal protuberance. Eup. p.
——— pain in left parietal protuberance. Lob. i.
——— pressing pain in, with drawing in the eyes, in the forenoon. Pod. p.
——— undulating pain in. Fluor. ac.
——— boring in left t. Trios.
——— in left t. stitches, periodic. Sang. c.
——— in left t. pain. Fluor. ac., Oxal. ac.
——— pressure in. Fluor. ac.
——— in the region of constructiveness, pain. Benz. ac.

Tension in the h., towards the right. Fluor. ac.
Throbbing in the h. Eup. p., Fluor. ac.
—— and pain in left side of head. Kalm. l.
—— above the right ear. Eup. p.
—— and bitter vomiting. Sang c.
—— worse by stooping. Sang. c.
—— worse by every motion. Sang. c.
Undulation in the head, painful. Fluor. ac.
Vertigo. Fluor. ac., Oxal. ac., Kalm. l., Lob. i., Sang. c., Trios.
—— with pain in head, and trembling of the body. Lob. i.
—— with nausea. Kalm. l., Lob. i., Sang. c.
—— with pains in head and limbs. Kalm. l.
—— with pain in head, on lying down. Oxal. ac.
—— on quickly turning the head and looking upwards. Sang. c.
—— when looking down. Kalm. l.
—— when stooping. Kalm. l.
—— with sens. of fulness over the eyes. Pod. p.
—— with darts of pain in forehead, obliging one to shut the eyes. Pod. p.
—— with inclination to fall forwards. Pod. p.
—— in the open air. Pod. p.
—— at midnight, with drowsiness. Trios.
Vertex, pain in. Oxal. ac., sang. c.
—— dull. Oxal. ac.
—— heaviness Oxal. ac.
—— pain as if bound with a cord. Kalm. l.
—— pain when rising in the morning. Pod. p.
—— heat in, with headache. Pod. p.
—— pressing in, disappears whilst walking. Sang. c.
Weakness of head, sens. of. Fluor. ac.
Headache, morning. Fluor. ac., Oxal. ac., Pod. p.
—— —— with flushed face. Pod. p.
—— forenoon. Fluor. ac., Pod. p.
—— at noon. Kalm. l.
—— every other morning, with nausea. Eup. p.
—— evening. Fluor. ac.
—— —— with tickling in the throat. Sang. c.
—— —— violent pressive pain, with heat of face. Lob. i.
—— afternoon, pain-like fulness in forepart of head. Sang. c.
Aggravated by stooping, headache. Fluor. ac.
—— by moving. Fluor. ac.
Head, exterior of.
Alopecia, (falling off of hair.) Fluor. ac.
Bones of temples, pain in. Fluor. ac.
—— jerking in, above right eyebrow. Fluor. ac.

Compression, on the right frontal protuberance. Fluor. ac.
Contraction on top of head towards the right, followed by pain under the right shoulder-blade. Fluor. ac.
Distension of veins on head. Sang. c.
——— on temples. Sang. c.
Fulness in the left parietal bone. Fluor. ac.
Itching on the head. Fluor. ac.
——— of scalp. Benz. ac.
Looseness of scalp on one side, on raising the eyes. Sang c.
Perspiration of head, during sleep, with coldness of the flesh while teething, in children. Pod. p.
Pressing, on the whole of the upper part of the head and spinal column, as if pressed together, in the morning. Benz. ac.
——— pain on left side of occiput. Fluor. ac.
——— dull in occiput towards the right. Fluor ac.
Soreness of head, with pain in spots. Sang. c.
——— of scalp, on being touched. Sang. c.

EYES AND SIGHT.

Angles, itching in. Benz. ac., Lob. i.
——— ——— left inner, violent. Fluor. ac.
——— ——— left eye. Lob. i.
——— ——— right inner, in evening. Fluor. ac.
Blotches, elevated, red, over the eyebrows. Fluor. ac.
Burning, in the eyes. Fluor. ac., Kalm. l., Lob. c.
——— in right eye. Sang. c.
——— itching in right eyebrow. Fluor. ac.
——— ——— in the internal canthis. Fluor. ac.
——— shooting pain at the bottom of the orbit. Fluor. ac.
Clearness of sight, with increased power of vision. Fluor. ac.
Cloudiness before the eyes. Kalm. l.
Drawing round the right eye in the evening. Fluor. ac.
Dilatation of pupils. Sang. c.
——— sens. of, in the eyes, with pain in the head. Pod. p.
Dimness of the eyes, and sens. as of hairs in them. Sang. c.
Diminished power of vision. Sang. c.
Enlarged circle of vision. Fluor. ac.
Eruption, scaly, with pricking sens. in eyebrows. Fluor. ac.
Glimmering, before the eyes, exactly in the point of vision, as if small points were continually moving before the eyes. Kalm. l.
——— ——— before the eyes. Sang. c.
Heat, under the eyes. Fluor. ac.
Heaviness of the eyes, with pain in top of head. Pod. p.
Inflammation of the eyes, the left one esp. Kalm. l.
——— sens. of. Fluor. ac.
Intolerance of light. Eup. p., Lob. c.

Itching in the eyes. Fluor. ac., Kalm. l.
——— and burning in the left eye, in the afternoon. Kalm. l.
——— burning in right eyebrow. Fluor. ac.
——— ——— near the right eye externally. Fluor. ac.
——— on upper eyelid. Fluor. ac.
——— in inner canthi. Fluor. ac.
——— painful in left eye, as if from a grain of sand. Fluor. ac.
——— and stinging when rubbed. Kalm. l.
Lachrymal Fistula. Fluor. ac.
Lachrymation, increased. Fluor. ac., Eup. p., Lob. c., Sang. c.
Light, jerking before the eyes, crossing itself like lightning, in the evening. Fluor. ac.
Objects, linear, appear larger and more distant. Oxal. ac.
Pleasant sensation as if the eyelids were wider opened, or the eyes more prominent. Fluor. ac.
Pain in both orbits, worse in left. Oxal. ac.
—— and soreness in the right eye. Lob. i.
—— and soreness in the left eyeball. Eup. p., Trios.
—— in right eye. Kalm. l., Sang. c.
—— in the eyes, making it painful to move them. Kalm. l.
—— in the eye-balls, and in the temples, with heat and throbbing of the temporal arteries. Pod. p.
Pressing in the eyes, with pains in the arms, hands, and lower extremities. Kalm. l.
——— above the right eye, sens. of. Kalm. l.
——— as if behind the right eyeball. Fluor ac.
——— in the upper part of the eyes, during walking. Oxal. ac. Lob. i.
——— pain about the eyes. Kalm. l.
——— pain in the left eye. Sang. c.
Pricking, sens. of, in eyebrows. Fluor. ac.
——— and burning in inner canthi. Fluor. ac.
Quivering, above the external canthus of the left eye. Fluor. ac.
——— externally on the right eye. Fluor. ac.
Redness of margins of lids, with glutinous secretion from the meibomian glands. Eup. p.
Ring, large, bright, on closing the eyes. Fluor. ac.
Smarting of inside of eyelids. Lob. i.
——— of eyes. Pod. p.
Soreness of eyeballs. Eup. p.
——— in the eyes, with smarting. Lob. c.
Sparklings, red, crossing each other, in the evening. Fluor. ac.
Spots, dark, floating before the eyes whilst reading. Fluor. ac.
Stiffness, sens. of, in the muscles around the eyes and eyelids. Kalm. l.
Stitches, acute in the eyes, towards evening. Kalm. l.
——— in right eye, in the morning. Kalm. l.

Stitches in right eye and violent pressure, with sens. of dimness and weakness. Kalm. l.
——— under the left eye. Kalm. l.
——— in upper eyelid. Sang. c.
Trembling, which disappears after opening the eyes. Fluor. ac.

EARS AND HEARING.

Beating under the ears, irregular. Sang. c.
Burning of ears, with redness of the cheeks. Sang. c.
Crackling in right ear, when drawing the fingers over the cheek. Sang. c.
Hearing, increased sensitiveness of, in the morning. Fluor. ac.
Humming in the ears, with determination of blood. Sang. c.
——— in left ear. Sang. c.
Itching in ears. Fluor. ac.
——— in left ear. Benz. ac., Fluor. ac.
Jerking behind the left ear. Fluor. ac.
Otalgia. See pain.
Pain, aching, in left ear. Lob. i.
—— in left ear, during pain in forehead. Sang. c.
—— behind the right ear, moving up towards the head. Fluor. ac.
—— in the right ear. Benz. ac., Fluor. ac.
—— in right side of the head, and in the leg. Kalm. l.
—— intermitting, Benz. ac.
—— pressing, in right ear. Fluor. ac.
—— Shooting. Benz. ac.
—— shooting, extending into left ear from a painful spot in the throat. Lob. i.
—— sticking, near the rim of the cartilage, of left ear. Elat.
Singing, sensation as if it would commence. Fluor. ac.
Sensitiveness of hearing, painful to sounds of a hammer. Sang. c.
Singing in the ears, with vertigo. Sang. c.
Stitches in right ear. Fluor. ac., Kalm. l.
——— severe in ears, followed by pain in the arms. Kalm. l.
——— slow, in left ear. Sang. c.
Tingling, excessive, in the ears. Kalm. l.

NOSE AND SMELLING.

Anosmia, (loss of smell.) Sang. c.
Coryza, flowing with sneezing. Eup. p., Kalm. l.
Dislike to the smell of syrups. Sang. c.
Eruption of pimples on the nose towards the right, between the root of the nose and eye. Fluor. ac.
——— of pimples, with inflamed base. Fluor. ac.
——— of pimples, filled with pus. Fluor. ac.
Heat in the nose, towards the right. Fluor. ac.
in the nose. Sang. c.

Inflammation of the nose, chronic, inside towards the tip. Fluor. ac.
Irritation, sens. of, in the left nostril. Fluor. ac.
Obstruction of nose. Kalm. l.
Pressing on ridge of nose. Kalm. l.
Polypus, nasal. Sang. c.
Redness of the nose, inside. Fluor. ac.
Smelling, increased sense of. Kalm. l.
Smell of roasted onions. Sang. c.
Sneezing. Eup. p., Kalm. l.
Tickling in the nose. Kalm. l.

TEETH AND GUMS.

Acrid, putrid taste, from the root of the right lateral incisor, on which there is fixed an artificial tooth. Fluor. ac.
Aggravation of pain in carious teeth, by drinking cold water. Sang. c.
Bleeding of the gums. Fluor. ac., Oxal. ac.
Caries of teeth. Fluor. ac.
Carious, molar tooth, pain in. Sang. c.
Cutting pain in teeth. Fluor. ac.
Digging pain in one of the lower incisors, towards the right. Fluor. ac.
Drawing pain in the left lower jaw. Fluor. ac.
Dull aching pains of the molar teeth of upper jaw. Oxal. ac.
—— pain, distressing, in the first molar tooth of the right upper jaw. Oxal. ac.
—— pain in incisor and eye-tooth. Kalm. l.
—— pressing in left molar teeth and temple. Lob. i.
Excoriation, painful near the first lower molar tooth, on the right side. Fluor. ac.
Grinding of the teeth at night. Pod. p.
Mucus dried on the teeth in the morning. Pod. p.
Looseness of the teeth. Sang. c.
Pressing, severe, in molar teeth, at night. Kalm. l.
Roughness of teeth. Fluor ac.
Shooting and thrilling pain in carious molar teeth of upper jaw. Sang. c.
Short pains in the teeth of the right side, in the evening. Kalm. l.
Teeth, pain from picking. Sang. c.
—— pain in hollow. Sang. c.
Upper teeth, pain in. Kalm. l., Sang. c.
—— carious teeth, pain, with headache in same side. Sang. c.
Warmth of teeth, sens. of. Fluor. ac.

FACE, LIPS AND MAXILLÆ.

Biting, involuntary, of lower lip at dinner. Fluor. ac.
Burning, on the outside of the right lower jaw, near the first or second molar tooth. Fluor. ac.
Chilliness, in left cheek, extending to the ear. Lob. i.
Compression in both zygomas with drawing downwards, towards the larynx. Fluor. ac.
Contractions, painful, spasmodic in both joints of the jaws. Fluor. ac.
Drawing, sens. of peculiar, extending from the right side of the mouth to the right eye. Lob. i.
——— pain in the right lower jaw bone. Fluor. ac.
——— in the entire left eye. Fluor. ac.
Dryness of the lips. Sang. c.
—— ——— and stiffness in the morning. Kalm. l.
Eruptions, vesicular, on the forehead. Lob. c.
——— small white, oblong, with itching and discharge, near the inner angle of the left eye. Fluor. ac.
Fissures, (cracks) in lips. Kalm. l.
Flushed face. Eup. p.
Fulness, sens. of, in face. Oxal. ac.
Gnawing, slight, pain in both sides of the lower jaw bone, near the angle. Fluor. ac.
Heat, first in the face, and afterwards in the left leg. Oxal. ac.
—— in the face. Fluor. ac., Oxal. ac., Lob. i.
—— ——— sudden flashes of. Kalm. l.
Itching in the face at night. Kalm. l.
——— on the right side of the face. Fluor ac.
——— slight, like pin prickings, on the right side of the face Fluor. ac.
Numbness, of the right joint of the lower jaw. Fluor. ac.
Pain, drawing, with rigidity, near the angle of the lower jaw. Oxal. ac.
—— as if something sharp pointed was moved about deep in the bone, behind the left eye, in the left nostril and forehead. Fluor. ac.
—— deep, posterior to the right eye, extending into the upper jaw. Fluor. ac.
——*ful* sensibility of the right upper jaw. Fluor. ac.
—— drawing, in the right lower jaw bone. Fluor. ac.
—— gnawing, slight, in both sides of the lower jaw, in the bone near the angle. Fluor. ac.
—— pressing, in the right side of the face between the eye and nose, in the afternoon. Kalm. l.
Perspiration of the face. Fluor. ac., Lob. i.
Redness of face. Oxal. ac., Eup. p.

Sallow sickly countenance. Eup. p.
Stiffness of the jaws. Sang. c.
Stinging in the bones of the jaws. Kalm. l.
Soreness, deep, superior and posterior to the left eye. Fluor. ac.
Warmth, sens. of, in the bone of the right upper jaw. Fluor. ac
——— sens. of, on lips. Fluor. ac.

MOUTH, THROAT, TASTE, PALATE AND TONGUE.

After-taste in mouth, of what has been eaten. Fluor. ac., Oxal. ac.
Burning, like a sore on the inside of the lower lip, towards the right, very near the edge. Fluor. ac.
——— violent in the fauces. Fluor. ac.
——— in the œsophagus. Sang. c.
——— in the throat. Lob. i.
——— sens. of, on tongue. Sang. c.
——— *prickling* in the throat. Lob. i.
——— ——— in the fauces and tongue. Lob. i.
——— in fauces, after drinking sweet things. Sang. c.
Chronic sore throat. Oxal. ac.
Choking. Fluor. ac.
Contraction of the œsophagus, as from below upwards, sens. of. Lob. i.
——— and tension, sens. of. Fluor ac.
Constriction in throat, with difficult deglutition. Fluor. ac.
Coldness of tongue. Fluor. ac.
Crawling on the tip of tongue. Sang. c.
Deglutition, difficult. Fluor. ac., Kalm. l.
——— painful. Fluor. ac., Oxal. ac., Benz. ac., Sang. c.
Dryness of the throat. Eup. p., Kalm. l., Lob. i., Lob. c., Pod. p., Sang. c.
——— of the left half of the palate, and roof of mouth. Fluor. ac.
——— of the mouth. Lob. i., Pod. p.
——— of tongue. Oxal. ac., Kalm. l., Pod. p.
——— of the fauces. Lob. i.
——— and rawness, beginning on the right side and spreading over the whole tongue. Sang. c.
Expansion, sens. of, in the posterior nares. Fluor. ac., Elat.
Furred Tongue. Fluor. ac., Eup. p.
——— ——— white. Eup. p., Kalm. l., Pod. p.
Greasy taste in mouth. Sang. c.
——— feeling in the mouth. Fluor. ac.
Goitre. Pod. p.
Heat, in the throat, alleviated by the inspiration of cold air. Sang. c.

Heat, sens. of, in mouth and fauces. Fluor. ac.
—— in the œsophagus. Benz. ac.
Hæmoptysis. Fluor. ac.
Inflammation of tongue and mouth. Oxal. ac.
———— of sublingual glands. Kalm. l.
Itching, (prickling) of tongue. Fluor. ac.
Lump, sens. of in pit of throat. Lob. i.
Mucus, collection of, in the mouth. Fluor. ac.
——— ejection of yellowish, from throat. Oxal. ac.
——— increased secretion of, from throat. Oxal. ac.
——— in the fauces, causing frequent hawking. Lob. i.
——— rattling of, in throat. Pod. p.
Odour, offensive, from the mouth. Pod. p.
Offensive breath at night. Pod. p.
Pain, drawing, in the right side of the throat extending to the ear. Lob. i.
—— in the mouth. Fluor. ac.
—— at the opening of the left eustachian tube. Fluor. ac.
—— severe, extending into the œsophagus. Fluor. ac.
Pharyngitis. Sang. c.
Pressing in the throat, and nausea, with stitches in the eyes. Kalm. l.
———— sens. of, as from a foreign body, in the whole course of the œsophagus. Lob. i.
Prickling in the throat. Lob. i.
———— sens. of, on tongue and roof of mouth. Sang. c.
Redness of tongue. Oxal. ac.
Salivation, increased. Kalm. l., Fluor. ac., Pod. p.
———— ———— viscid. Fluor. ac., Lob. i.
Scalding, sens. of, in mouth. Fluor. ac.
Scraping in the throat. Kalm. l.
———— day and night, which excites a cough. Kalm. l.
———— sens. of, in the lower part of the entrances of the fauces, towards the left. Fluor ac.
Skin, paleness of, mucous membrane of mouth. Eup. p.
—— whiteness and peeling off of. Fluor. ac.
Stitches in the tongue. Kalm. l.
——— left side. Sang. c.
Sores in the corners of the mouth. Eup. p.
Soreness, in the mouth. Fluor. ac., Oxal. ac., Pod. p.
——— of fauces. Eup. p., Benz. ac., Fluor. ac., Lob. i., Lob. c., Oxal. ac.
——— of palate. Benz. ac.
——— of tongue. Benz. ac., Sang. c.
——— of roof. Benz. ac.
——— of throat, extending below the pharynx. Fluor. ac., Lob. i.
———— of throat. Lob. i., Pod. p., Sang. c., Trios.

Soreness of left side when swallowing liquids, worse in the morning. Pod. p.
Swallowing (see deglutition.)
Swelling of tongue. Oxal. ac.
——— sens. of, in the throat, with pain and aphonia. Sang. c.
Sticking, sens. of, in mouth. Fluor. ac.
Taste in the mouth and pharynx,
—— acid. Fluor. ac., Oxal. ac.
—— acrid. Kalm. l.
—— —— on rinsing the mouth. Oxal. ac.
—— bitter. Elat., Kalm. l.
—— disagreeable. Fluor. ac., Lob. i., Lob. c.
—— ——— flat. Fluor. ac.
—— of fried liver at night. Pod. p.
—— foul, acrid, from the root of a tooth. Fluor. ac.
—— foul. Pod. p.
—— greasy. Fluor. ac., Sang. c.
—— slimy, in mouth. Sang. c.
—— inky, in the evening. Fluor. ac.
—— intolerable. Fluor. ac.
—— insipid. Eup. p.
—— pungent. Lob. i.
—— saltish, in the morning. Fluor. ac.
—— sour. Oxal. ac., Fluor. ac.
—— sweetish, in the throat at night. Fluor. ac.
—— loss of. Sang. c.
Tenderness of tongue. Oxal. ac.
Tightness of tongue. Oxal. ac.
Tingling in the salivary glands. Kalm. l.
Tumour, ulcerated, in the left side of the mouth, behind the last molar tooth. Benz. ac.
Ulcers on the tongue, extensive fungoid. Benz. ac.
——*ated* tumour behind the last molar tooth. Benz. ac.
—— painful, small, toward the right, in the corner of the upper and lower jaw. Fluor. ac.
—— in throat. Sang. c.
Viscid saliva, at night previous to an attack of diarrhœa. Fluor. ac.
—— mucus in mouth. Fluor. ac.
White furred tongue. Eup. p., Kalm. l.
—— —— —— with loss of appetite. Sang. c.
Yellow furred tongue. Eup. p.

APPETITE, HUNGER AND THIRST.

Adipsia, Oxal. ac.
After-taste, of food, worse in afternoon. Fluor. ac.
After-meals, food turns sour. Pod. p.

After meals bitter eructations. Fluor. ac.
Anorexia. Trios.
Appetite, increased. Oxal. ac., Fluor. ac., Trios.
——— diminished. Fluor. ac., Lob. c.
——— loss of. Eup. p., Oxal. ac., Lob. i., Sang. c.
——— want of. Eup. p.
——— voracious. Fluor. ac., Sang. c.
Aversion to coffee. Fluor. ac.
——— to water. Oxal. ac.
Bulimia, Fluor. ac.
Desire for particular things,
——— ice cream. Eup. p.
——— for something sour. Pod. p.
Eructations, in gen., acid. Pod. p.
——— with pyrosis and flatulency. Fluor. ac.
——— fluid, with burning sens. Lob. i.
——— bitter after dinner. Fluor. ac.
——— disgusting, with inclination to vomit. Fluor. ac.
——— nauseating, with inclination to vomit. Fluor. ac.
——— with sickness of stomach. Fluor. ac.
——— with discharge of flatulency, per anum. Oxal. ac.
——— sour. Fluor. ac.
——— of wind. Elat., Fluor. ac., Lob. i., Oxal. ac., Sang. c.
——— tasteless. Eup. p.
——— spasmodic. Sang. c.
Heart-burn. Lob. i., Pod. p., Sang. c.
——— with running of water in the mouth. Lob. i.
Hiccough, (see singultus.)
Hunger, excessive. Fluor. ac.
——— increase of. Oxal. ac., Fluor. ac.,
——— satisfied by a small quantity of food, followed by nausea and vomiting. Pod. p.
Nausea, in gen. Elat., Eup. p., Fluor. ac., Kalm. l., Lob. i., Lob. c., Sang. c., Trios.
——— attended by,
——— chills. Sang. c.
——— desire to vomit. Elat., Fluor. ac., Lob. i., Sang. c.
——— eructations. Fluor. ac.
——— general heat. Fluor. ac.
——— headache. Fluor. ac., Kalm. l., Sang. c.
——— pressing in the throat, and stitches in the eyes. Kalm. l.
——— pyrosis. Fluor. ac.
——— salivation extreme. Sang. c.
——— vertigo. Fluor. ac.
——— violent, shivering and shaking of the upper parts of the body. Lob. i.
——— vomiting, with perspiration and expectoration. Eup. p.

Nausea vomiting. Fluor. ac., Trios.
—— ——— of food. Eup. p.
—— from stooping. Sang. c.
—— preceding nettle rash. Sang. c.
Pyrosis, (see water-brash.)
Qualmishness of the stomach,
———— with sickness. Oxal. ac.
———— from odours, the smell of food cooking, &c., Eup. p.
Regurgitation of food. Pod. p.
Singultus, (hiccough.) Benz. ac., Lob. i., Sang. c.
——— with flow of saliva. Lob. i
Satiety, from a small quantity of food. Pod. p., Fluor. ac.
Thirst. Trios.
—— moderate during fever. Pod. p.
—— unusual. Oxal. ac.
—— violent. Oxal. ac.
—— at night. Fluor. ac.
—— ——— for something cold. Eup. p.
—— for cold water. Eup. p., Lob. c.
—— towards evening. Pod. p.
Thirstlessness. Oxal. ac.
Vomiting, Eup. p., Fluor. ac., Lob. i., Oxal. ac., Pod. p., Sang. c., Trios.
——— of clear viscid fluid, with coagulated white pieces. Fluor. ac.
——— of bitter water. Sang. c.
——— of bile. Eup. p.
——— ——— with pain in the epigastrium. Eup. p.
——— copious. Lob. i.
——— distressing disposition to. Eup. p.
——— of hot frothy mucus. Pod. p.
——— of food. Eup. p., Pod. p.
——— ——— an hour after a meal. Pod. p.
——— ——— immediately after drinking. Eup. p.
——— ——— preceded by thirst. Eup. p.
——— ——— with nausea. Eup. p.
——— ——— of food with putrid taste and odour. Pod. p.
——— with profuse perspiration. Lob. i.
——— with perspiration and expectoration. Eup. p.
——— with cold perspiration of the face. Lob. i.
——— with great weakness, but good appetite, shortly after. Lob. i.
——— with craving of food. Sang. c.
——— with nausea, and fulness in the head. Pod. p.
——— *preceded by*, great anxiety. Sang. c.
——— ———— slight pressure to stool. Sang. c.
——— in the morning, on rising to stool. Trios.

Vomiturition, with pain in the epigastrium, and drawing in the calves of the legs. Trios.
Voracity, voracious appetite. Eup. p., Fluor. ac.
Water-brash, Pod. p., Fluor. ac., Oxal. ac.
——— every evening. Oxal. ac.
——— with acid eructations, and passage of flatulency. Fluor. ac.
——— with much emission of flatulency, and pressing downwards. Oxal. ac.

STOMACH, ABDOMEN, ETC.

Burning, gnawing and eructations in st. Oxal. ac.
——— *pain in st.* and throat. Oxal. ac.
——— ——— towards the back, as if inflamed. Lob. i.
Cramp in abd. Elat.
——— in abdomen, changing from one place to another. Sang. c.
Colic, flatulent. Elat.
——— with retraction of the abdominal muscles. Pod. p.
——— with torpor of the liver. Sang. c.
——— *a* pictonum. Elat.
——— in the morning, followed by a diarrhœal stool. Sang. c.
——— attended by diarrhœa. Elat., Sang. c.
Digging pain in the abdomen, with pain in the sacrum. Sang. c.
Distension of abdomen, with shortness of breathing. Lob. i.
——— in the evening, with escape of flatus from the vagina. Sang. c.
Drawing, slight, with cutting in abdomen. Sang. c.
Faintness, sens. of, in region of the navel, with desire to draw a deep breath, relieved by bandaging, and after eating. Fluor. ac.
Fulness, in region of *stomach*, with constriction in the throat, and frequent eructations. Fluor. ac.
——— in stomach, sens. of. Eup. p.
——— in right hypochondrium, with flatulence. Pod. p.
——— in right *hypochondrium*, with pain and soreness. Sang. c. Pod. p.
Grasping, in abdomen.
Heat, in stomach. Eup. p., Fluor. ac.
——— in *abdomen*, sens. of. Benz. ac., Pod. p.
——— in *stomach*, before meals, followed by heaviness after meals, and worse during exercise. Fluor. ac.
Indurations, in abdomen. Sang. c.
Inflammation of the abdl. viscera. Sang. c.
Jerking, in abd., left side. Fluor. ac.
Liver, *inflammation*, of. Pod. p., Sang. c
——— chronic. Pod. p., Sang. c.
——— ——— with costiveness. Sang. c.

Liver, torpor and atony of. Sang. c.
—— hot, streaming towards, from the breast. Sang. c.
Pain, in *abdomen* severe. Lob. i.
—— —————— across. Kalm. l.
—— —————— left side of, just below the short ribs. Benz. ac.
—— —————— left side of, in the region of the spleen. Fluor. ac.
—— —————— left side of, and left arm, pressing in the evening. Fluor. ac.
—— —————— worse after eating. Lob. i.
—— —————— *right side* of, followed by a pain in the glutæus muscle. Kalm. l.
—— —————— with heat, in the evening. Trios.
—— in the *bowels*, attended at first by coldness, then followed by warmth. Pod. p.
—— —————— cramp-like, with retraction of the abdl. muscles, morning and evening. Pod. p., Elat.
—— in the *bowels*, dull. Elat.
—— —————— at daylight in the morning, relieved by lying on the side and bending forwards, and external warmth; aggravated by lying on the back. Pod. p.
—— in the *colon* ascending. Pod. p.
—— —————— transverse, followed by diarrhœa. Pod. p.
—— just above the hips, hindering respiration. Fluor. ac.
—— in right hypochondrium, dull. Elat., Lob. i.
—— in left hypochondrium, aggravated by pressure, and lying on the left side. Pod. p.
—— in hypochondriæ, severe and continued, with vertigo and debility. Pod. p.
—— over the crest of right ilium, dull, aching, pressing, extending around the back, and deep into the pelvis. Oxal. ac.
—— *liver*, in region of, right side. Kalm. l.
—— *navel*, in the region of, during diarrhœa. Fluor. ac.
—— *sharp*, above the right groin, preventing motion, in the latter months of pregnancy. Pod. p.
—— *shooting*, as from wind. Fluor. ac.
—— in *scrobiculus*, pressive, violent, like a heavy weight, at intervals of 15 minutes. Oxal. ac.
—— —————— increased by drinking water, and turning in bed. Trios.
—— —————— dull. Elat.
—— spleen, in region of, extending to the hips. Fluor. ac.
—— in stomach. Oxal. ac.
—— —————— burning. Oxal. ac.
—— —————— excruciating. Oxal. ac.
—— —————— after eating water melon, fish, &c. Fluor. ac.
Oppression in scrobiculus, at night. Trios.

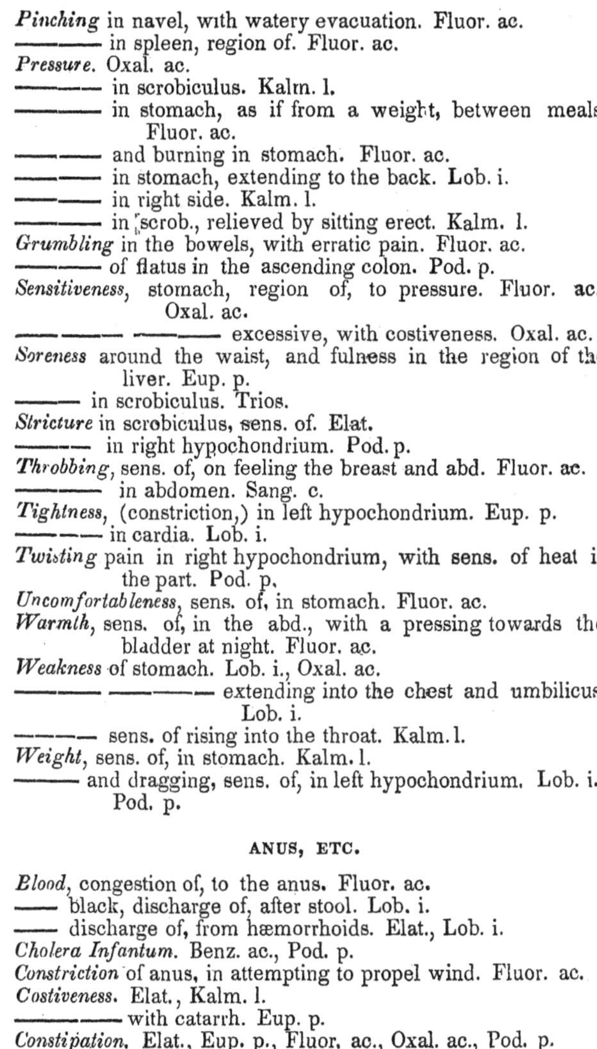

Pinching in navel, with watery evacuation. Fluor. ac.
——— in spleen, region of. Fluor. ac.
Pressure. Oxal. ac.
——— in scrobiculus. Kalm. l.
——— in stomach, as if from a weight, between meals. Fluor. ac.
——— and burning in stomach. Fluor. ac.
——— in stomach, extending to the back. Lob. i.
——— in right side. Kalm. l.
——— in scrob., relieved by sitting erect. Kalm. l.
Grumbling in the bowels, with erratic pain. Fluor. ac.
——— of flatus in the ascending colon. Pod. p.
Sensitiveness, stomach, region of, to pressure. Fluor. ac., Oxal. ac.
——— ——— excessive, with costiveness. Oxal. ac.
Soreness around the waist, and fulness in the region of the liver. Eup. p.
——— in scrobiculus. Trios.
Stricture in scrobiculus, sens. of. Elat.
——— in right hypochondrium. Pod. p.
Throbbing, sens. of, on feeling the breast and abd. Fluor. ac.
——— in abdomen. Sang. c.
Tightness, (constriction,) in left hypochondrium. Eup. p.
——— in cardia. Lob. i.
Twisting pain in right hypochondrium, with sens. of heat in the part. Pod. p.
Uncomfortableness, sens. of, in stomach. Fluor. ac.
Warmth, sens. of, in the abd., with a pressing towards the bladder at night. Fluor. ac.
Weakness of stomach. Lob. i., Oxal. ac.
——— ——— extending into the chest and umbilicus. Lob. i.
——— sens. of rising into the throat. Kalm. l.
Weight, sens. of, in stomach. Kalm. l.
——— and dragging, sens. of, in left hypochondrium. Lob. i., Pod. p.

ANUS, ETC.

Blood, congestion of, to the anus. Fluor. ac.
—— black, discharge of, after stool. Lob. i.
—— discharge of, from hæmorrhoids. Elat., Lob. i.
Cholera Infantum. Benz. ac., Pod. p.
Constriction of anus, in attempting to propel wind. Fluor. ac.
Costiveness. Elat., Kalm. l.
——— with catarrh. Eup. p.
Constipation. Elat., Eup. p., Fluor. ac., Oxal. ac., Pod. p.

Diarrhœa, bilious. Elat., Pod. p.
——— inclination to. Fluor. ac., Oxal. ac.
——— with pain in region of navel. Oxal. ac.
——— painful, with screaming and grinding of the teeth, in children, during dentition. Pod. p.
——— during the day 4 or 5 natural stools. Sang. c.
——— morning, in. Eup. p., Kalm. l., Pod. p.
——— evening, in. Sang. c.
——— every other day. Fluor. ac.
——— preceded by coryza, catarrh, or pain in the breast. Sang. c.
——— *Chronic*, worse in the morning. Pod. p.
Dysentery. Sang. c.
——— bilious. Elat.
Evacuations, alvine.
——— bilious. Elat.
——— copious, of thin stools, without pain. Trios.
——— copious, pappy, preceded by discharge of flatulence, and accompanied by pain in the region of navel. Fluor. ac.
——— copious, pappy, with blueness under the eyes. Pod. p.
——— ——— in the morning. Fluor. ac.
——— desire for, ineffectual. Fluor. ac., Sang. c.
——— difficult, hard and dry. Pod. p.
——— disagreeable smell of. Fluor. ac.
——— fetid, watery, white stools, very copious and exhausting in infants, with urine of a deep red colour. Benz. ac.
——— free, twice a day. Fluor. ac., Oxal. ac.
——— frothy. Elat.
——— hasty pressure for a passage, like in diarrhœa. Fluor. ac.
——— ineffectual desire for. Fluor. ac.
——— inclination to. Kalm. l., Oxal. ac.
——— involuntary, of fluid fæces mixed with blood. Oxal. ac.
——— loose. Fluor. ac., Kalm. l.
——— ——— at noon. Kalm. l.
——— lumpy. Fluor. ac.
——— muco-gelatinous, small with flatulence and pain in sacrum. Pod. p.
——— pappy. Fluor. ac., Lob. i., Oxal. ac., Pod. p.
——— ——— thick and short. Oxal. ac.
——— protracted. Fluor. ac.
——— purging. Eup. p., Sang. c.
——— ——— with smarting heat in anus. Eup. p.
——— soft. Kalm. l., Lob. i.

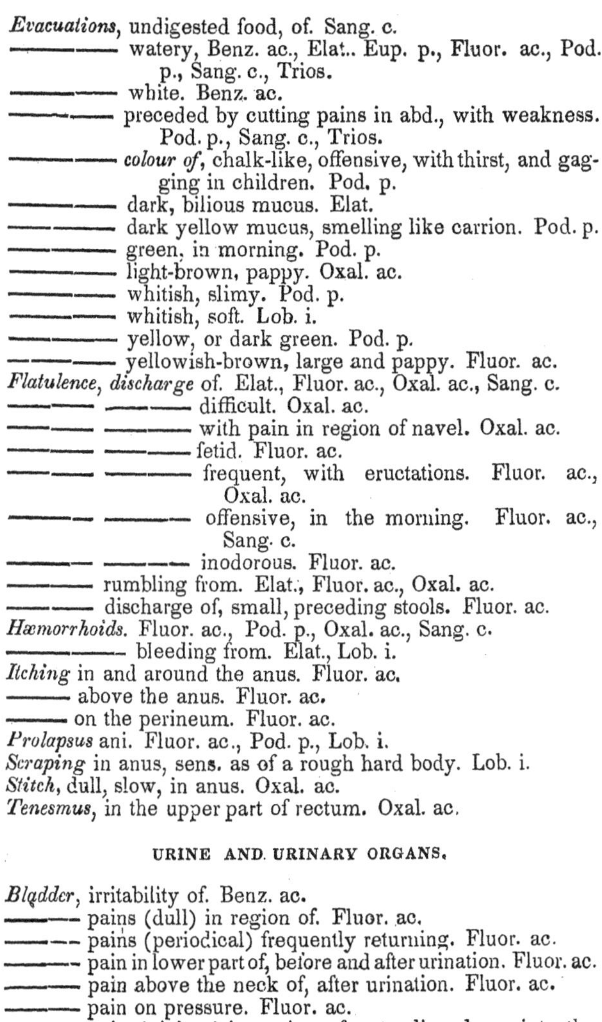

URINE AND URINARY ORGANS.

Bladder, pressure on, with a sensation of warmth in the abd. Fluor. ac.
Enuresis. Pod. p.
Inguina, pain in region of, both sides. Fluor. ac.
——— right, burning pain in region of. Fluor. ac.
Nephritic colic, with high coloured and strongly scented urine. Benz. ac.
Urethra, aching pain in. Lob. i.
——— intolerable burning in, during urination, and 5 minutes after. Fluor. ac.
Urine, discharge of, copious. Benz. ac., Eup. p., Oxal. ac., Sang. c.
——— ——— diminished. Fluor. ac., Oxal. ac., Lob. i., Pod. p.
——— ——— *frequent*. Fluor. ac., Pod. p., Sang. c.
——— ——— ——— with strong pressing. Benz. ac.
——— ——— ——— nocturnal, during pregnancy. Pod. p.
——— ——— hot, scalding of deep red colour and strong odour. Benz. ac.
——— ——— *increased in quantity* and frequency. Kalm. l. Lob. i.
——— ——— ——— but not in frequency. Benz. ac., Elat.
——— ——— involuntary. Pod. p.
——— ——— nocturnal, (copious.) Sang. c.
——— ——— painful. Benz. ac.
——— ——— profuse, of light colour. Oxal. ac.
——— ——— with loose *cloudy sediment*. Lob. i.
——— ——— with purple sediment. Fluor. ac.
——— ——— with red sediment. Lob. i.
——— ——— with pink sediment, and a small brown crystal. Lob. i.
——— ——— whitish sediment. Fluor. ac.
Urine, colour of, dark brown, scanty with whitish clay like sediment. Eup. p.
——— ——— high, (scanty.) Eup. p.
——— ——— high, like brandy with strong urinous odour. Benz. ac.
——— ——— light. Fluor. ac., Oxal. ac., Eup. p.
——— ——— red, (deep) with copious red sed. Lob. i.
——— ——— red, (deep) heavy and without sed. Benz. ac.
——— ——— yellow. Kalm. l.
Urine, odour of, acrid. Fluor. ac.
——— ——— fragrant. Fluor. ac.
——— ——— offensive. Fluor. ac.
——— ——— pungent and strong. Benz. ac., Fluor. ac.

SEXUAL. (MALE.)

Chancre, with high coloured and strongly scented urine. Benz. ac.
Glans penis, (left side of,) thrilling sens. almost painful, extending into the urethra, and ending in a sens. of tickling and itching. Benz. ac.
Itching, in the sulcus behind the corona glandis. Benz. ac.
Seminal emissions, during sleep. Fluor. ac., Sang. c.
Sexual desire, diminished. Fluor. ac.
——— excessive. Oxal. ac.
——— erections, on lying down followed by pains in the testicles. Oxal. ac.
——— *increased.* Fluor. ac., Oxal. ac.
——— ——— with erection during sleep. Fluor. ac., Oxal. ac.
Smarting of the *frænum præputii.* Benz. ac., Lob. i.
Spermatic chords, sens. of fulness in. Fluor. ac.
Syphilis. Benz. ac.
Syphilitic rheumatism. Benz. ac.
Testicles, jerking in, and spermatic chord. Oxal. ac.
——— pain in, and spermatic chord, worse on right side. Oxal. ac.
——— *left* drawing through to the abdl. ring. Fluor. ac.
——— — occasional stitches, and drawing through to the abdl. ring, and spermatic chord. Fluor. ac.

SEXUAL. (FEMALE.)

Abdominal pains, as if the menses would appear. Sang. c.
——— ——— at night. Sang. c.
Abortion. Sang. c.
After pains, with strong bearing down. Pod. p.
——— with heat and flatulency. Pod. p.
Amenorrhœa. Sang. c., Kalm. l.
Climacteric disorders. Sang. c.
Dysmenorrhœa. Sang. c.
Itching of mons veneris. Eup. p.
Labia, swelling of, during pregnancy. Pod. p.
Leucorrhœa, yellowish in the morning. Kalm. l.
——— of thick transparent mucus. Pod. p.
——— with constipation and bearing down in genitals. Pod. p.
Menses, too early appearance of. Pod. p., Sang. c.
——— painful. Kalm. l.
——— retarded. Fluor. ac., Kalm. l., Pod. p.
——— suppression of. Kalm. l., Lob. i., Pod. p.
——— thick, coagulated. Fluor. ac.

Ovaria, pain in region of. Pod. p.
——— numb, aching pain in region of *left* o. with heat running down the left thigh. Pod. p.
Pregnancy, during inability to lie on abd. in early part of. Pod. p.
———— swelling of labia. Sang. c.
Prolapsus uteri. Pod. p.
———— symptoms of, after parturition, with rumbling of flatus in region of ascending colon. Pod. p.
Uterine hæmorrhage. Lob. i.? Sang. c.

BACK AND LOINS.

Bruised, sens. in back, from loins to shoulders. Oxal. ac.
Creeping of cold, from lower part of spine upward. Oxal. ac.
Heat, strong, extending from the centre of the dorsal region to the loins. Fluor. ac.
Itching, violent with small pimples on both shoulders and back. Fluor. ac.
Jerking, in sacrum. Fluor. ac.
Lameness, in small of back, in the evening. Kalm. l.
Numbness, and weakness in back and limbs. Oxal. ac.
——— sens. of in sacrum. Oxal. ac.
Pain, aching. Kalm. l.
—— ——— in os sacrum. Fluor. ac.
—— acute, in back, gradually extending down into the thighs. Oxal. ac.
—— bruised, in os sacrum and lumbar region. Fluor. ac.
—— ——— as if, in back. Eup. p.
—— constant, in spine, with heat and burning. Kalm. l.
—— deep seated, in the back below the point of shoulder blades, more towards the left. Fluor. ac.
—— ———— in the left lumbar region, at night. Fluor. ac.
—— ———— in loins, with soreness from motion. Eup. p.
—— dull, in region of kidneys. Benz. ac.
—— paralytic in small of back, at night, with dulness and pain in head. Kalm. l.
—— rheumatic, in the back, from stooping. Trios.
—— ——— in nape, shoulders and arms. Sang. c.
—— ——— in right shoulder, worse in the forenoon. Sang. c.
—— ——— in right arm and shoulder, worse at night, and inability to raise the arm. Sang. c.
—— ——— sudden in shoulder joint. Sang. c.
—— severe, in left shoulder. Sang. c.
—— ——— in every motion, in upper part of shoulder joint. Sang. c.
—— sharp, in the three superior dorsal vertebræ, extending through to the shoulder blades. Kalm. l.
—— shooting, downwards from the loins to the limbs. Oxal. ac.
—— sticking, in lower part of the left shoulder blade. Kalm. l.

Pain, sticking, in region of right kidney. Lob. i.
—— in the back. Sang. c.
—— ———— and lower extremities. Eup. p.
—— ———— sometimes high up, near the shoulder blades, sometimes deeply seated in the region of kidneys. Fluor. ac.
—— ———— small of, when walking or standing. Pod. p.
—— in loins, with sens. of coldness, worse at night and from motion. Pod. p.
—— in loins. Lob. i.
—— ———— and stiffness. Trios.
—— ———— region of, towards the right, after rising. Oxal. ac.
—— ———— left side. Trios.
—— in shoulders. Sang. c.
—— in right shoulder, and upper part of right arm, worse at night on turning in bed. Sang. c.
—— right shoulder, on top of. Sang. c.
—— ———— from lying on it. Trios.
—— shoulder blades, in. Kalm. l.
—— ———— under, with chill. Sang. c.
—— ———— under the point of right. Fluor. ac., Pod. p.
—— between the shoulders, with soreness. Pod. p.
—— in sacrum, and bowels. Sang. c.
—— ———— from lifting. Sang. c.
—— ———— alleviated by bending forwards. Sang. c.
—— ———— in the morning. Oxal. ac.
Pressing, below the left shoulder, in the evening. Kalm. l.
Pricking, burning, itching, near the os coccygis, towards the right. Fluor. ac.
Sensation, as if the spinal column would break, with an anterior convexity. Kalm. l.
Stitches, under the left arm. Kalm. l.
Weakness, in small of back. Eup. p.

LARYNX.

Aphonia, with swelling in the throat. Sang. c.
Dryness, (chronic) in the throat, with sens. of swelling in the larynx, and expectoration of thick mucus. Sang. c.
Expectoration, of hard mucus in lumps, and watery running from the nose, with sneezing. Oxal. ac.
———— of thick yellow mucus from the throat. Oxal. ac.
———— of thick mucus. Sang. c.
———— easy. Lob. i., Sang. c.
———— ———— of a gray, smooth, unctuous matter, with putrid salty taste. Kalm. l.
———— ———— extending through the abdomen. Kalm. l.
———— ———— extending to the legs. Pod. p.

Cough, disposition to, with dyspnœa. Eup. p.
—— dry. Pod. p.
—— excited by a scraping in the larynx. Kalm. l.
—— with coryza, then diarrhœa. Sang. c.
—— dry, awaking one from sleep, ceasing with discharge of flatus upwards and downwards. Sang. c.
—— with expectoration. Sang. c.
—— continual, severe, without expectoration, with pain in the breast, and circumscribed redness of the cheeks. Sang. c.
—— following and preceding measles. Eup. p.
—— hacking, in the evening. Eup. p.
—— hectic, from suppressed int. fever. Eup. p.
—— loose hacking. Pod. p.
—— nocturnal, loose. Eup. p.
—— slight. Sang. c.
—— —— from tickling in the larynx and trachea. Oxal. ac., Sang. c.
—— —— frequent, especially whilst eating. Sang. c.
—— troublesome, and almost constant dry, hacking. Benz. ac., Lob. i.
—— violent, with soreness in the chest. Eup. p.
—— tormenting, with expectoration, and circumscribed redness of the cheeks. Sang. c.
—— with soreness and heat in the bronchia. Eup. p.
—— with flushed face and tearful eyes. Eup. p.
—— with easy expectoration of a gray, smooth unctuous matter, with a putrid, salt taste. Kalm. l.
—— aggravated in the evening. Sang. c.
Hooping Cough, with costiveness and loss of appetite. Lob. i., Pod. p.
Hoarseness. Oxal. ac.
———— slight, with sneezing and without accompanying catarrhal symptoms. Benz. ac.
———— with roughness of the voice. Eup. p.
Influenza. Sang. c., Eup. p.
Irritability, increased, of larynx. Fluor. ac.
———— a peculiar feeling, between tickling and smarting. Lob. i.
Lump, sens. of, in pit of throat impeding respiration and de glutition. Lob. i.
Mucus, sens. of, in larynx. Oxal. ac.
—— secretion of, increased. Oxal. ac.
—— ———— diminished. Oxal. ac.
Pain in larynx, as if in the cartilage inducing deglutition. Fluor. ac.
Sore throat, chronic. Oxal. ac.
Soreness, sens. of, in larynx while coughing, slightly. Fluor. ac.

Tickling in larynx, with a sens. of sticking, the larynx feels swelled. Oxal. ac.

CHEST AND HEART.

Aching in region of heart. Fluor ac.
Asthma. Lob. i., Sang. c., Benz. ac.?
Beating, audible, of the heart. Trios.
Burning feeling in the breast, passing upwards. Lob. i.
——— and pressing in the breast, then heat through the abdomen. Sang. c.
Drawing, feeling of, in left breast, from the nipple to the axilla. Lob. i.
Eruption, of a thin brownish crust, on the areola of nipple. Fluor. ac.
Grating sens. of, in the chest, at every deep inspiration. Eup. p.
Hydrothorax. Fluor. ac. Sang. c.
Inability to lie down on the left side. Eup. p.
Irritation, painful, of the pulmonary organs, with heat in the chest. Eup. p.
Itching, on the left breast and right side of the nose after smelling, Fluor. ac.
——— on the right nipple and around it. Fluor. ac.
——— severe, on the breast with small soft pimples, in summer. Fluor. ac.
Jerking, painful, in the heart. Fluor. ac.
Oppression of the chest. Kalm. l., Lob. i.
——— ——— with sens. of swelling in the throat. Kalm. l.
——— ——— with dyspnœa, dulness of head, and nausea. Kalm. l.
——— ——— towards the right side. Oxal. ac.
——— ——— on reclining, accompanied by trembling in the lower extremities. Fluor. ac.
——— ——— upper part of, not relieved by deep inspiration. Fluor. ac.
——— of respiration accelerated, with sens. as if a deeper inspiration was required. Lob. i.
——— ——— with dull and distressing pain in the lower part of sternum, and at each side. Lob. c.
——— ——— with sticking pains, on taking a long breath. Lob. c.
——— requiring deep inspiration. Lob. i.
——— with pain in the chest. Fluor. ac.
Palpitation of the heart. Sang. c., Kalm. l.
——— ——— with a clucking sens. rising up into the throat. Pod. p.

Palpitation of the heart, from exertion or mental emotion. Pod. p.

—— —— immediately after lying down at night. Oxal. ac.

Pain in the chest. Lob. i.

—— —— with cough and expectoration. Sang. c.

—— —— with dry cough. Sang. c.

—— —— with periodic cough. Sang. c.

—— —— increased by deep inspiration. Lob. i., Pod. p.

—— —— after dinner, when walking. Lob. i.

—— about the third rib, on the right side midway between the sternum and the side. Benz. ac.

—— about the third, fourth, and fifth dorsal vertebræ. Lob. i.

—— in the right side of the back, about midway between the tenth vertebra dorsalis and the side. Benz. ac.

—— in the left side, about the sixth rib, increased by deep inspirations, and by bending the body to either side. Benz. ac.

—— under the middle of sternum. Lob. i.

—— aching, under the left breast. Eup. p.

—— burning, in a small spot under the right breast. Lob. i.

—— —— sticking, in the left side of the chest, momentary. Fluor. ac.

—— boring, violent, through the back under the right shoulder. Lob. i.

—— deep penetrating, in the posterior part of the left side, about the sixth rib. Benz. ac.

—— deep seated, in the left side and in the right shoulder. Eup. p.

—— —— in region of the heart. Lob. i.

—— drawing, slight, between the scapulæ. Lob. i.

—— rheumatic, between the scapulæ. Lob. i.

—— numb, the whole length of the scapula, increased by breathing. Sang. c.

—— pressing, in the breast and back. Sang. c.

—— —— in the region of the heart. Sang. c.

—— —— at the left side of the lower part of sternum. Lob. i.

—— —— in the last rib towards the right, near the spine. Fluor. ac.

—— —— in the middle of the chest. Fluor. ac.

—— pricking, in left lung. Lob. c.

—— sharp, at the lower part of the sternum, passing through to the spine or lower part of right shoulder-blade. Elat.

—— sharp lancinating, in the left lung, coming on suddenly. Oxal. ac.

—— sharp shooting, in the left lung and heart, extending to the epigastrium. Oxal. ac.

Pain, slight, close to the right nipple. Fluor. ac.
—— —— under the left breast. Trios.
—— slowly shooting, in the right side of the chest, about the seventh rib. Sang. c.
—— ———— in the left side of the chest near the axilla. Sang. c.
—— ———— under the sternum. Sang. c
—— sore, in the left side of chest, as if beneath the skin, felt only while moving, and accompanied by a similar pain in the left shoulder, in the evening. Fluor. ac.
—— —— in the left side of chest, similar to the last, in the morning on rising. Fluor. ac.
—— sticking, in the region of the heart. Pod. p.
—— as if a stitch would appear deep in the left side of the chest, behind the heart. Fluor. ac.
—— shifting, constantly, but is most permanent in the region of the heart.
—— like a stitch, from the left side of the chest to the groin, increased by respiration. Fluor. ac.
—— violent, in the heart, extending from behind and below anteriorly. Oxal. ac.
Pressing, and heaviness, constant, in the whole of the upper part of the chest, with difficult breathing. Sang. c.
———— in the centre of the sternum in the afternoon, in the evening a pressing pain in the middle of the chest. Fluor. ac.
Respiration, difficult, (dyspnœa,) (chronic,) with a sens. of a lump in the pit of throat, impeding deglutition and respiration. Lob. i.
———— difficult, frequently returning in the afternoon and evening. Fluor. ac.
———— —— attended with perspiration and anxious countenance, with sleepiness. Eup.p.
———— —— obliging the patient to lie with the head and shoulders very high. Eup. p.
———— —— with constrictive pain in the larynx and wheezing. Oxal. ac.
———— —— there seems to be an impediment in pit of throat and upper part of chest, at the same time itching pimples on the back and pain in the chest below the point of shoulder-blade. Fluor. ac.
———— abdominal. Lob. i.
———— deep, as if the breast within and below was full, in the forenoon during sitting and writing Fluor. ac.
———— great difficulty of holding the breath. Lob. i.

Respiration, short inspiration and slow expiration. Lob. i.
———— wheezing. Fluor. ac.
Inspiration, deep. Lob. i.
———— —— inclination to. Pod. p.
———— —— relieving a pressive pain in the epigastrium Lob. i.
Sensation in chest as if strained by lifting. Kalm. l.
———— in chest as if the heart was ascending to the throat. Pod. p.
Shortness of breath. Pod. p.
Snapping, in the right lung, like breaking a thread, aggravated by deep inspiration. Pod. p.
Sneezing, with gaping and flatulent eructation. Lob. i.
Soreness, continual, in the heart. Fluor. ac.
———— in the chest. Eup. p., Fluor. ac.
———— sens. of, in larynx. Oxal. ac.
Stitches, in the left breast, worse while walking. Oxal. ac.
———— in the lower part of chest. Kalm. l.
———— small, in the side. Fluor. ac.
Sticking, under the ribs, to the left of the ensiform cartilage, in the evening. Fluor. ac.
Suffocation, sens. of, when first lying down at night. Pod. p.
Streaming, hot burning, in the right breast, drawing downwards towards the liver. Sang. c.
Tickling, slight, on taking a deep breath, under the lower part of the sternum. Lob. i.
Tightness, general, of the chest, with short and difficult breathing. Lob. i.
———— of the chest, with heat in the forehead. Lob. i.
Uneasiness, about the heart. Fluor. ac.

UPPER EXTREMITIES.

Aching, in the right elbow joint. Fluor. ac.
———— in the left elbow, in the evening. Fluor ac.
———— in the left index finger. Fluor. ac.
Arthritis. Elat., Eup. p., Oxal. ac.
Bruised, and benumbed sens. in the right upper arm and shoulders, on awaking, after lying on the left side. Fluor. ac.
Burning of the palms. Sang. c.
———— around the bone of the right middle finger, with an itching stinging in the skin. Fluor. ac.
Cracking of the joints of the elbows, frequent, strong. Kalm. l.
Drawing, in the right wrist and forearm. Fluor. ac.
Eruption of large and small vesicles in groups, with sens. of itching on the ulnar side of the right thumb, and the radial side of the index finger, leaving behind them dry scurfy spots. Fluor. ac.
Heaviness, in the right arm, in the morning on awaking. Fluor. ac.

Heat, in the palms of the hands, sometimes with moisture. Eup. p.

—— in the palm of the right hand. Fluor. ac.

Itching, severe, on the right shoulder. Fluor. ac.

—— —— with occasionally a severe stitch in the skin, changing from the top of one shoulder to the other, in the evening. Fluor. ac.

—— violent, on the left shoulder, in the afternoon, on the back in the evening, where small pimples arise. Fluor. ac.

—— —— on the right index finger, with eruption of small vesicles. Fluor. ac.

Jerking, electric, along the left radius to the thumb, which moves involuntarily. Fluor. ac.

—— in the left thumb, occasionally extending to the middle of the forearm. Fluor. ac.

—— slowly, repeated, burning, in the end of the little finger. Fluor. ac.

Knicking, and cracking of the joints. Benz. ac.

Lameness, of right arm. Fluor. ac.

—— —— with pricking sens. Fluor. ac.

—— of right hand. Fluor. ac.

Lividity of the hands, in pneumonia. Sang. c.

Numbness, sleep, of left hand and forearm, in the morning. Fluor. ac.

—— sens. of, in the left hand, extending to the forearm. Fluor. ac.

—— with jerking and lameness in the left arm, in the morning. Fluor. ac.

—— and weakness in the head and hands. Fluor. ac.

—— and rigidity, in the fingers of the right hand. Fluor. ac.

Pain, aching, in the bones of the left forearm, towards the middle. Fluor. ac.

—— burning, pricking, in the left shoulder blade. Fluor. ac.

—— —— and jerking, in the whole left arm, as if a slow electric shock was passing through the nerves. Fluor. ac.

—— cramp-like, from the elbow down to the middle of the arm. Kalm. l.

—— contused, as if, in the ends of several fingers. Fluor. ac.

—— cutting, on the second joint of the left middle finger. Sang. c.

—— deep penetrating, first in the right, then in the left arm. Fluor. ac.

—— drawing, on the inner side of the left arm, transitory. Kalm. l.

—— dull, in the right shoulder, forearm and hand, extending to the fingers. Elat.

Pain, numb, in the forearms and hands. Fluor. ac.
—— —— in ball of right thumb. Sang. c.
—— pressing, in the right arm, and a constriction in the left side of the neck, in the morning. Fluor. ac.
—— —— in the left arm, just above the elbow. Fluor. ac.
—— rheumatic, in the bones of the left arm, from elbow to shoulder, with lameness. Fluor. ac.
—— —— in the arms and hands. Sang. c.
—— —— in right arm and shoulder, worse at night. Sang. c.
—— —— in the right forearm, in the evening. Sang. c.
—— —— slight, in the right shoulder joint. Lob. i.
—— —— in shoulder joint. Sang. c.
—— —— severe, in the right elbow joint. Lob. i.
—— shifting, as from the hand to the opposite arm, then in the heart, &c. Benz. ac.
—— severe in the hand, with aching in the arm, when lying warm and quiet in bed Sang. c.
—— —— as from a bile, in the right palm, near the index finger. Sang. c.
—— slight pinching, in the middle of the left forearm. Fluor. ac.
—— sudden jerking, in the left shoulder, in the bone. Fluor. ac.
—— sharp sticking, in the muscular parts of the thumb. Elat.
—— —— in the fingers of the left hand out to their extremities. Elat.
—— in the joints of the fingers of the right hand. Benz. ac.
—— about the right wrist and finger joints. Fluor. ac.
—— in the right elbow joint and left side. Fluor. ac.
—— in the right elbow joint. Lob. i.
—— in the right shoulder joint of short duration, and extending towards the fingers, as if air was passing down. Fluor. ac.
—— in the first joint of the right little finger. Fluor. ac.
—— in the right hand. Kalm. l.
—— in the right arm. Kalm. l.
—— in the right metacarpus, from exposure to cold. Fluor. ac.
—— in the right upper arm, in the bone towards the elbow, passing to the left arm, in the afternoon. Fluor. ac.
—— in the left arm, above the elbow, following the pains in the right side. Fluor. ac.
—— in the left shoulder, beneath the skin, and in the left side of the chest. Benz. ac.
—— in the left wrist, as if palsied. Kalm. l.
—— in the left index finger, as if in the bone. Fluor. ac.
—— in the left hand, close to the wrist in the palm. Kalm. l.
—— in all the fingers of the left hand. Kalm. l.
—— in the muscles of the right arm, only when touched. Lob. i.

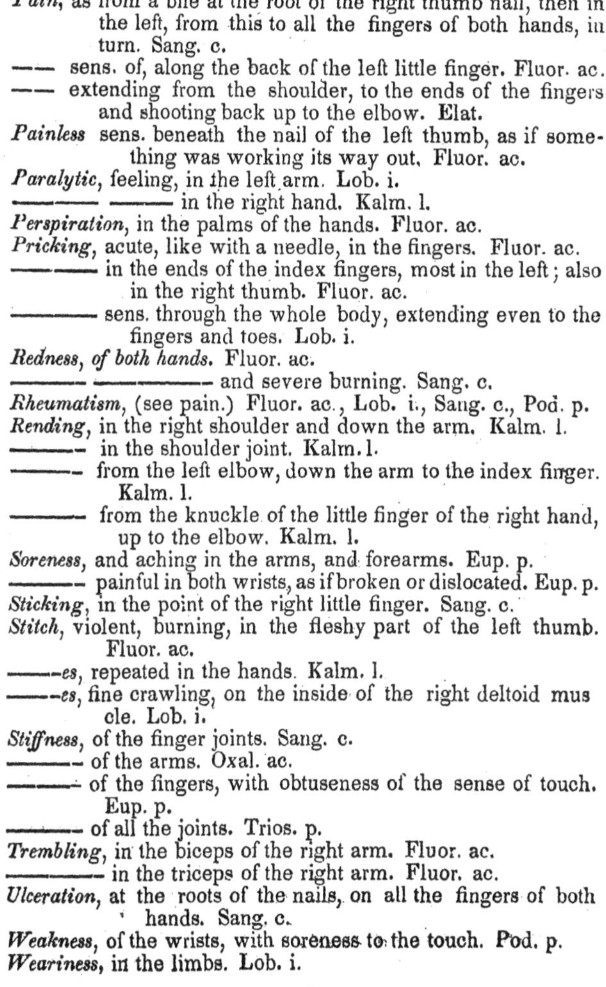

Pain, as from a bile at the root of the right thumb nail, then in the left, from this to all the fingers of both hands, in turn. Sang. c.

—— sens. of, along the back of the left little finger. Fluor. ac.

—— extending from the shoulder, to the ends of the fingers and shooting back up to the elbow. Elat.

Painless sens. beneath the nail of the left thumb, as if something was working its way out. Fluor. ac.

Paralytic, feeling, in the left arm. Lob. i.

—— —— in the right hand. Kalm. l.

Perspiration, in the palms of the hands. Fluor. ac.

Pricking, acute, like with a needle, in the fingers. Fluor. ac.

—— in the ends of the index fingers, most in the left; also in the right thumb. Fluor. ac.

—— sens. through the whole body, extending even to the fingers and toes. Lob. i.

Redness, *of both hands*. Fluor. ac.

—— —— and severe burning. Sang. c.

Rheumatism, (see pain.) Fluor. ac., Lob. i., Sang. c., Pod. p.

Rending, in the right shoulder and down the arm. Kalm. l.

—— in the shoulder joint. Kalm. l.

—— from the left elbow, down the arm to the index finger. Kalm. l.

—— from the knuckle of the little finger of the right hand, up to the elbow. Kalm. l.

Soreness, and aching in the arms, and forearms. Eup. p.

—— painful in both wrists, as if broken or dislocated. Eup. p.

Sticking, in the point of the right little finger. Sang. c.

Stitch, violent, burning, in the fleshy part of the left thumb. Fluor. ac.

——*es*, repeated in the hands. Kalm. l.

——*es*, fine crawling, on the inside of the right deltoid muscle. Lob. i.

Stiffness, of the finger joints. Sang. c.

—— of the arms. Oxal. ac.

—— of the fingers, with obtuseness of the sense of touch. Eup. p.

—— of all the joints. Trios. p.

Trembling, in the biceps of the right arm. Fluor. ac.

—— in the triceps of the right arm. Fluor. ac.

Ulceration, at the roots of the nails, on all the fingers of both hands. Sang. c.

Weakness, of the wrists, with soreness to the touch. Pod. p.

Weariness, in the limbs. Lob. i.

LOWER EXTREMITIES.

Arthritic inflammation of the left knee, and the right elbow. Eup. p.
Anthritis, (see pain.)
Aching, slight, in the left hand and fingers, and in the posterior part of the left leg, towards the heel, with jerking in the heel. Kalm. l.
——— of the limbs, worse at night. Pod. p.
——— in the tarsal bones of the right foot. Kalm. l.
Beaten, sens. as if, in the calves of the legs. Eup. p.
Burning, of the hands and feet, in the night. Sang. c.
——— in the skin on the inner side of the thighs of a female. Eup. p.
——— in the soles of the feet and in the palms of the hands, forenoon. Sang. c.
——— in the soles of the feet, worse at night. Sang. c.
——— sens. in the sole of the right foot. Fluor. ac.
——— stitches, in the morning, under the soles of both feet. Fluor. ac.
Coldness, and stiffness in the feet. Trios. p., Pod. p.
——— feeling of, in the knees, as if they were blown upon by a cold wind. Benz. ac.
Cracking, in the knee joints from motion. Pod. p.
Cramp, in the calf of the leg on awaking from a restless sleep. Lob. i.
——— like feeling, in the left gastrocnemius. Lob. i.
——— —— in the hollow of the left foot. Lob. i.
——— and pain, in the calf of the left leg. Sang. c.
Crawling, sens. of, in the sole of the right foot. Fluor. ac.
Drawing, in the calves and into the instep, worse right than left. Sang. c.
——— and shrinking, sens. of, in the legs and pricking in the soles of the feet. Trios. p.
Eruption, of red inflamed spots, like the beginning of blood biles, in different places on the body. Kalm. l.
Flagging of the muscles of the left thigh, as if they were falling off the bone. Eup. p.
Heat, in the sole of the right foot. Fluor. ac.
——— in the soles of the feet in the morning. Eup. p.
Heaviness, and stiffness of the knees as after a long walk. Pod. p.
Itching, on various parts of the body and extremities, yielding an agreeable feeling on being scratched, but followed by a burning. Benz. ac.
——— in the bend of the right knee, in the afternoon. Kalm. l.
——— in the left instep. Fluor. ac.

Itching, excessive and burning, of red spots, about the size of a pea, in the region of the knee. Kalm. l.
Knicking and cracking of the joints. Benz. ac.
Lividity of the nails and fingers. Oxal. ac.
——— coldness, and almost complete loss of motion in the legs. Oxal. ac.
Lameness and stiffness in the lower extremities. Oxal. ac.
——— in the left hip. Fluor. ac.
——— in the right hip and lower extremity when walking. Eup. p.
——— in right foot, and a dull aching pain in the os femoris, tibia and fibula. Fluor. ac.
——— sens. of, like a sprain in the right ankle-joint. Fluor. ac.
Numbness, in the right knee-joint. Fluor. ac.
——— of left leg. Fluor. ac.
——— in the shins, in the afternoon. Kalm. l.
——— of the limbs as if asleep. Kalm. l.
——— in the calves of the legs. Trios. p.
Perspiration of the feet in the evening. Pod. p.
Pain, aching, in the right hip. Eup. p.
—— ——— in the left hip, then in the thigh, next in the knees then in the toes. Benz. ac.
—— ——— in the right ankle-joint, with a sensation of swelling. Oxal. ac.
—— acute, pricking, in the ends of the toes of the right foot. Fluor. ac.
—— bruise-like, of the thigh. Fluor. ac.
—— ——— alternating with burning and pressure in the breast. Sang. c.
—— ——— in the left hip-joint, whilst walking, but worse on rising from a seat. Sang. c.
—— burning, in the right instep. Fluor. ac.
—— ——— itching, in the back part of the thigh. Fluor. ac.
—— ——— shooting, as if in the nerve, from the right hip downwards. Fluor. ac.
—— ——— violent, in all the toes. Fluor. ac.
—— contracting, violent, in the external tendon of the left knee. Oxal. ac.
—— deep-seated, below the right knee. Fluor. ac.
—— drawing, in the left leg and foot. Fluor. ac.
—— ——— in the calf of the right leg. Fluor. ac.
—— ——— in the right ankle-joint, in the evening during a walk, spreading gradually over the whole leg, and causing lameness. Fluor. ac.
—— frequent, here and there in the limbs, continually changing from one place to another. Kalm. l.

Pain, frequent in the muscles of the extremities, and also in the head, with dulness, vertigo, &c. Kalm. l.
—— ——— sliding, in the hollow of the left knee. Oxal. ac.
—— peculiar, along the outside of the left leg, frequently repeated. Kalm. l.
—— penetrating, on the outside of the left knee. Fluor. ac.
—— ——— under and behind the left external malleolus after sleeping. Trios.
—— pressing, in the fleshy part of the thigh. Fluor. ac.
—— ——— in the left shin, and in the muscles of the right arm. Kalm. l.
—— ——— in the left foot. Fluor. ac.
—— ——— in the whole body. Kalm. l.
—— ——— on the exterior middle part of the thigh, with constrictive feeling in the head. Lob. i.
—— rheumatic, on the inside of left knee. Eup. p.
—— ——— in the left hip. Sang. c.
—— ——— in the limbs. Sang. c.
—— ——— on the inside of right thigh. Sang. c.
—— severe, in the left knee, on the outside, disappears after friction. Fluor. ac.
—— ——— in all the toes of left foot, except the large one. Fluor. ac.
—— ——— in the hollow of the right knee and in the calf of the leg, with dyspnœa, preceded by a sticking pain in the right index finger. Kalm. l.
—— ——— in the tendo achillis close to the os calcis, when supporting a part of the weight of the body on the left foot. Benz. ac.
—— sharp, in the right ankle-joint. Oxal. ac.
—— ——— in the outer and upper portion of the left foot. Pod. p.
—— ——— in the left ankle, during the time it supports the weight of the body in walking. Benz. ac.
—— ——— shooting, coming on suddenly and lasting about 15 minutes. Oxal. ac.
—— ——— ——— on the instep of the right foot. Oxal. ac.
—— shooting, and also dull aching pains in the left thigh, in the course of the sciatic nerve, extending to the instep and extremities of the toes. Elat.
—— spasmodic, violent, in the left posterior iliac region Lob. i.
—— sprain-like, in the left ankle-joint during walking. Fluor. ac.
—— sprain-like, in the feet and hands, occasionally. Kalm. l.
—— sticking, in the right hip joint. Oxal. ac.

Pain, sticking in the right ankle Sang. c.
—— tearing, violent, in the fibula from below up to the knee-joint. Lob. i.
—— —— in the right knee, from below upwards, followed by a quick very transient pressing pain in the left temple. Fluor. ac.
—— violent, in the left foot. Kalm. l.
—— —— slightly burning, quick nervous pain, proceeding from the bladder down to the right thigh. Fluor. ac.
—— in both lower extremities, especially in the knees, with pain in the right shoulder and in the left arm. Kalm. l.
—— in both legs and in the left arm in the evening. Kalm. l.
—— in the thighs, legs and knees, worse from standing. Pod. p.
—— in the right thigh and ankle, shifting. Benz. ac.
—— in the right hip. Fluor. ac.
—— in the right tendo achillis, and in the region of the heart. Benz. ac.
—— in the left tendo achillis, after leaving the right. Benz. ac.
—— on the right knee, inside of. Fluor. ac.
—— in the right external ankle. Fluor. ac,
—— in the right knee, extending to the instep and toes. Elat.
—— in the right knee. Trios. p.
—— in the right ischiatic nerve. Fluor. ac.
—— in the corns of right foot. Fluor. ac.
—— in the left leg whilst sitting. Lob. i.
—— over the left hip, with soreness in a spot not larger than a pea. Eup. p.
—— in the left glutæi muscles, passing round in front of the trochanter major, accompanied by great sensitiveness. Eup. p.
—— in the foot, increased by standing on it. Eup. p.
—— in the left instep. Fluor. ac.
—— and weakness in the left hip, like rheumatism from cold. Pod. p.
—— in the left femur, inner condyle of. Fluor. ac.
—— in the gastrocnemii. Benz. ac.
—— in the left knee, leg and foot. Pod. p.
—— in the left knee and foot, and also in the right foot. Kalm. l.
—— in the bend of left knee, followed by severe pain in left index finger, and right foot. Kalm. l.
—— in the left foot. Kalm. l.
—— in the left elbow, arm and knee, in the morning. Kalm. l.
—— in the left foot, with headache. Sang. c.

Pain, and soreness of the upper part of the left foot with increased sensibility of the left big toe. Eup. p.
—— in the toes. Benz. ac.
—— in the large joints of great toes, with slight tumefaction and redness. Benz. ac.
—— in the great toe, of an arthritic nature. Elat.
—— in the first joint of the left great toe, suddenly moving to the corresponding joint of the right one. Eup. p.
—— in the toes of the right foot in the first joints. Fluor. ac.
Painful excoriation on the second toe of the left foot. Fluor. ac.
Paralytic feeling in the left arm. Lob. i.
—— weakness, slight, of the whole side. Pod. p.
Pressure and lameness, with pain in the forearm. Fluor. ac.
—— in the left shin and shoulder, and also in the left arm, followed by pressing in the right shoulder and arm. Kalm. l.
Pricking, in the soles of the feet. Eup. p.
Rheumatism, (see pain) acute, inflammatory and arthritic. Sang. c.
—— inflammatory of the right knee, with extreme pain and swelling. Lob. i.
Rheumatic pain in the limbs. Sang. c.
Stiffness and general soreness of the lower extremities when rising to walk. Eup. p.
—— of the knees. Sang. c.
—— —— when attempting to rise. Trios.
—— and tightness in the bend and sides of the knees. Sang. c.
—— of all the joints of the upper as well as of the lower extremities. Trios.
—— remarkable, in the lower extremities, with slight coldness, and tingling sens. Trios.
—— of the joints of the toes, ankles and knees when lying. Trios.
—— of the limbs, and rheumatic pains with headache. Sang. c.
Sticking in the soles of the feet. Kalm. l., Lob. c.
—— as from a needle in the instep, in the morning in bed. Sang. c.
Stinging, in the toes. Kalm. l.
—— in the great toe of the left foot. Kalm. l.
Stitches, suddenly attacking the hip bones of the right side in the evening. Kalm. l.
—— on the lower part of the knee, outside, in the evening. Kalm. l.
—— acute, on the right hip bone. Fluor. ac.

A stitch, passing perpendicularly upwards through the right great toe, followed by a burning, then again a stitch, and afterwards appearing in the left great toe. Benz. ac.

Soreness and pain on motion in the left hip, worse in the morning on getting out of bed. Fluor. ac.

——— in the muscles of the thighs. Fluor. ac.

——— and swelling of both feet, when standing on them. Eup. p.

——— and aching of the lower limbs. Eup. p.

Swelling, acute, of the joints of the extremities. Sang. c.

——— dropsical, of the feet and ankles. Eup. p.

A Twitch in the left deltoid muscle, followed by one in the right after lying down in bed. Oxal. ac.

Uneasiness in limbs and feet. Oxal. ac.

Weakness of the limbs, with pains in the sacrum. Sang. c.

——— of the joints, especially of the knees. Pod. p.

Weariness in the limbs. Lob. i., Kalm. l.

ERRATA.

Page 13, 7th line from bottom, for "Pharmocopœias" read Pharmacopœias.
15, 12th " top, for "graminivrous" read graminivorous.
18, 11th " top, for "fœtid" read fetid.
19, 4th, 10th, and 16th from bottom, for "achilles" read achillis.
21, 20th line from bottom, for "physcian" read physician.
23, 17th " " for "fœtid" read fetid.
35, 9th " " for "continues" read continue.
37, 4th " " for "this ceases" read these cease.
40, 15th " " for "not gums or alveolar process" read not in the gums or alveolar processes.
40, 16th " top, for "jaws" read jaw.
43, 20th " top, for "rincing" read rinsing.
48, 5th " bottom, for "disagreable" read disagreeable.
51, 14th " top for "stiches" read stitches.
52, 19th " " for "rincing" read rinsing.
53, 18th " " for "stiches" read stitches.
58, 4th " " for "a week" read the week.
59, 10th " " for "hand" read hands.
59, 17th " " after "wrist" read and.
61, 8th " " for "glutei" read glutæi.
62, 11th " " for "achilles" read achillis.
67, 18th " bottom, for "glutei" read glutæi.
72, 13th " top, for "the perennial and barks" read perennial and the barks.
72, 2d " bottom, for "eues" read neues.
72, 16th " " for "chalices" read calices.
77, 6th " " for "œsophages" read œsophagus.
77, 20th " " for "ceteris" read cæteris.
114, 13th " top, for "rincing" read rinsing.
127, 14th " bottom, for "was" read were.
136, 17th " " for "alleopathists" read allœopathists.
137, 20th " " for "wineglassfull" read wineglassful.
139, 21st " " for "developement" read development.
143, 7th " top, for "glutei" read glutæi.
151, 14th " bottom, "dispondancy" read despondency.
152, 15th " top for "wineglassfull" read wineglassful.
154, 10th " " for "Sweedish" read Swedish.
158, 14th " " for "cervicle" read cervical.
163, 10th " bottom, for "stiches" read stitches.
164, 20th " " for "gluteus" read glutæus.
167, 11th " " for "stiches" read stitches.
172, 15th " " for "calix" read calyx.
177, 6th " " for "cotemporaneous" read contemporaneous.
179, 14th " " for "euphorbia" read euphorbium.
196, 14th " top, for "climactric" read climacteric.
207, 11th " bottom, for "hemoptysis" read hæmoptysis.
208, 18th " " for "hemorrhoids" read hæmorrhoids.
210, 2d " top, for hypochondriæ" read hypochondria.
212, 8th " " for "voraceous" read voracious.
219, 8th " " for "filliform" read filiform.
228, 11th " " for "disposion" read disposition.
251, 4th " " for "emectic" read emetic.
248, 2d " bottom, for "later" read latter.
248, 7th " " for "illi" read ilii.

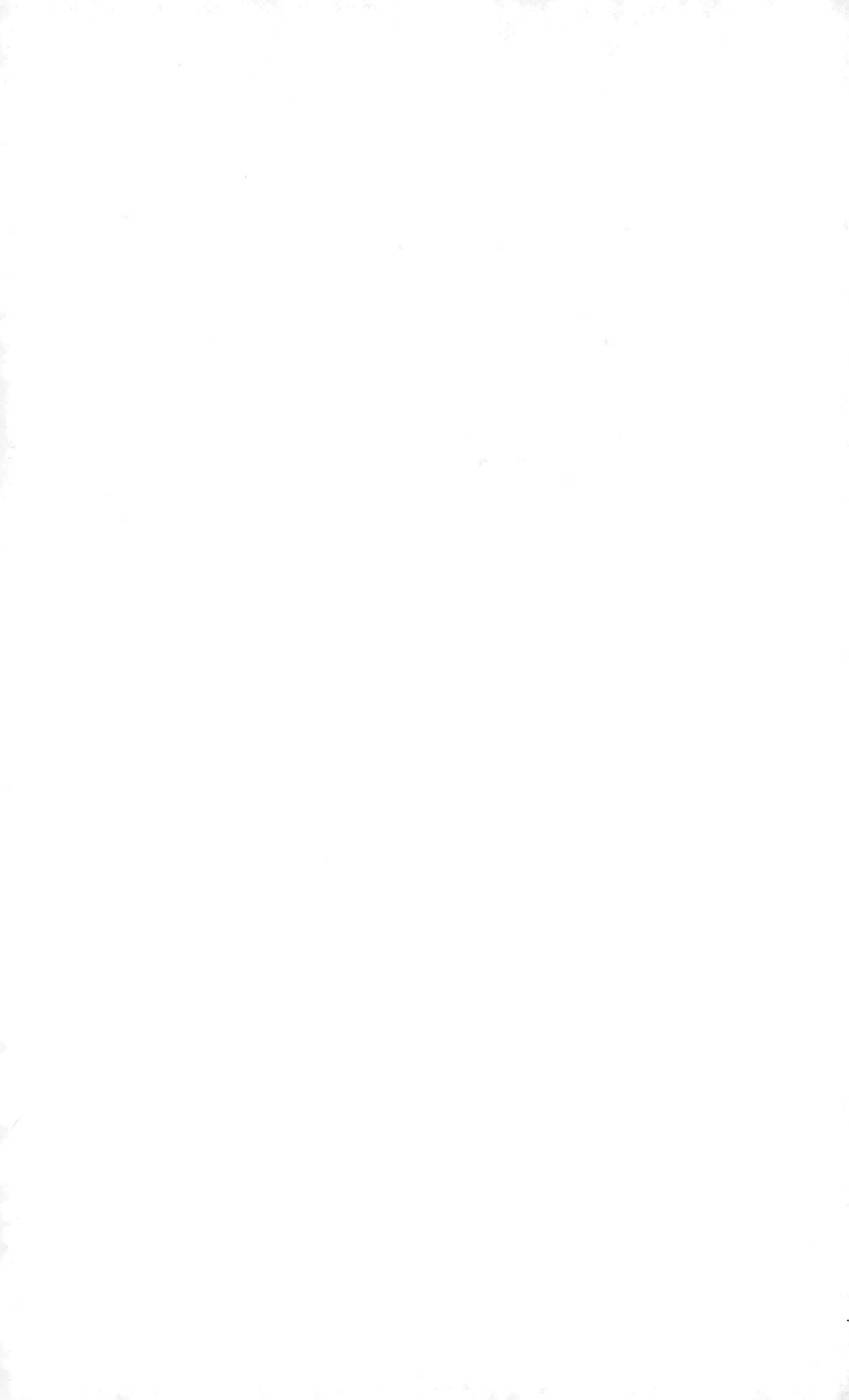

www.ingramcontent.com/pod-product-compliance
Lightning Source LLC
LaVergne TN
LVHW010210110826
845151LV00004B/1042

* 9 7 8 1 4 2 5 5 2 8 8 6 7 *